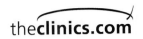

PHYSICAL MEDICINE AND REHABILITATION CLINICS

OF NORTH AMERICA

The Child and Adolescent
Athlete

GUEST EDITOR
Brian J. Krabak, MD, MBA

CONSULTING EDITOR
George H. Kraft, MD, MS

May 2008 • Volume 19 • Number 2

SAUNDERS

An Imprint of Elsevier, Inc.
PHILADELPHIA   LONDON   TORONTO   MONTREAL   SYDNEY   TOKYO

W.B. SAUNDERS COMPANY
A Division of Elsevier Inc.

1600 John F. Kennedy Blvd. • Suite 1800 • Philadelphia, Pennsylvania 19103

http://www.theclinics.com

PHYSICAL MEDICINE AND REHABILITATION
CLINICS OF NORTH AMERICA
May 2008
Editor: Debora Dellapena

Volume 19, Number 2
ISSN 1047-9651
ISBN 1-4160-5819-2
978-1-4160-5819-9

The ideas and opinions expressed in *Physical Medicine and Rehabilitation Clinics of North America* do not necessarily reflect those of the Publisher. The Publisher does not assume any responsibility for any injury and/or damage to persons or property arising out of or related to any use of the material contained in this periodical. The reader is advised to check the appropriate medical literature and the product information currently provided by the manufacturer of each drug to be administered to verify the dosage, the method and duration of administration, or contraindications. It is the responsibility of the treating physician or other health care professional, relying on independent experience and knowledge of the patient, to determine drug dosages and the best treatment for the patient. Mention of any product in this issue should not be construed as endorsement by the contributors, editors, or the Publisher of the product or manufacturers' claims.

Physical Medicine and Rehabilitation Clinics of North America (ISSN 1047-9651) is published quarterly by Elsevier Inc., 360 Park Avenue South, New York, NY 10010-1710. Months of publication are February, May, August, and November. Business and Editorial Offices: 1600 John F. Kennedy Blvd., Suite 1800, Philadelphia, PA 19103-2899. Customer Service Office: 6277 Sea Harbor Drive, Orlando, FL 32887-4800. Periodicals postage paid at New York, NY and additional mailing offices. Subscription price per year is $197.00 (US individuals), $308.00 (US institutions), $99.00 (US students), $240.00 (Canadian individuals), $394.00 (Canadian institutions), $135.00 (Canadian students), $277.00 (foreign individuals), $394.00 (foreign institutions), and $135.00 (foreign students). Foreign air speed delivery is included in all *Clinics* subscription prices. All prices are subject to change without notice. POSTMASTER: Send address changes to *Physical Medicine and Rehabilitation Clinics of North America*, Elsevier Periodicals Customer Service, 6277 Sea Harbor Drive, Orlando, FL 32887-4800. **Customer Service: 1-800-654-2452 (US). From outside of the United States, call 1- 407-563-6020. Fax: 1-407-363-9661. E-mail: JournalsCustomer Service-usa@elsevier.com.**

Physical Medicine and Rehabilitation Clinics of North America is indexed in *Excerpta Medica, Index Medicus, Cinahl,* and *Cumulative Index to Nursing and Allied Health Literature.*

Printed in the United States of America.

CONSULTING EDITOR

GEORGE H. KRAFT, MD, MS, Alvord Professor of Multiple Sclerosis Research; Professor, Rehabilitation Medicine; and Adjunct Professor, Neurology, University of Washington, School of Medicine, Seattle, Washington

GUEST EDITOR

BRIAN J. KRABAK, MD, MBA, Clinical Associate Professor, University of Washington Sports and Spine Rehabilitation; Children's Hospital and Regional Medical Center, Departments of Rehabilitation, Orthopaedics and Sports Medicine, Team Consultation, University of Washington, Seattle, Washington

CONTRIBUTORS

ERIC ALEXANDER, MD, Resident, Rehabilitation Medicine, University of Washington, Seattle, Washington

DANIELLE B. CAMERON, BA, Clinical Research Coordinator, Department of Orthopaedic Surgery, Children's Hospital of Philadelphia, Philadelphia, Pennsylvania

MICHAEL W. COLLINS, PhD, Assistant Director, University of Pittsburgh Medical Center Sports Medicine Concussion Program, Department of Orthopaedic Surgery, University of Pittsburgh Medical Center, Pittsburgh, Pennsylvania

SHEILA A. DUGAN, MD, Assistant Professor, Department of Physical Medicine and Rehabilitation; and Department of Preventive Medicine, Rush Medical College, Chicago, Illinois

THEODORE J. GANLEY, MD, Director of Sports Medicine, Department of Orthopaedic Surgery, Children's Hospital of Philadelphia; Assistant Professor of Orthopaedic Surgery, The University of Pennsylvania School of Medicine, Philadelphia, Pennsylvania

GERALD A. GIOIA, PhD, Director, Safe Concussion Outcome Research and Education (SCORE) Program, Associate Professor, Department of Pediatrics, George Washington University School of Medicine and Children's National Medical Center, Washington, District of Columbia; and Department of Psychiatry, George Washington University School of Medicine and Children's National Medical Center, Washington, District of Columbia

KATIE GOOSSEN, BS, Medical student, Department of Orthopedic Surgery, Medical College of Wisconsin, Milwaukee, Wisconsin

MATTHEW GRADY, MD, FAAP, Staff physician, Department of Orthopedics, Children's Hospital of Philadelphia, Philadelphia, Pennsylvania

TROY HENNING, MD, Resident, Rehabilitation Medicine, University of Washington, Seattle, Washington

ANNE Z. HOCH, DO, MD, PT, Associate Professor, Sports Medicine Center; Director, Women's Sports Medicine Program, Department of Orthopaedic Surgery, Cardiovascular Center, Medical College of Wisconsin, Milwaukee, Wisconsin

BRIAN J. KRABAK, MD, MBA, Clinical Associate Professor, University of Washington Sports and Spine Rehabilitation; Children's Hospital and Regional Medical Center, Departments of Rehabilitation, Orthopaedics and Sports Medicine, Team Consultation, University of Washington, Seattle, Washington

TRICIA KRETSCHMER, BS, Kinesiology student, University of Wisconsin–Milwaukee, Milwaukee, Wisconsin

GERARD A. MALANGA, MD, Associate Professor of Physical Medicine and Rehabilitation, University of Medicine and Dentistry, New Jersey Medical School, Newark; Director, Sports Medicine, Department of Orthopedic Surgery, Mountainside Hospital, Montclair; and Director, Department of Rehabilitation Medicine, Pain Management Center, Overlook Hospital, Summit, New Jersey

LYLE MICHELI, MD, Director, Division of Sports Medicine, Boston Children's Hospital, Boston; Associate Clinical Professor of Orthopaedic Surgery Harvard Medical School, Boston, Massachusetts

ANGELA H. NIPPERT, PhD, Associate Professor, Term Faculty, Department of Kinesiology and Health Sciences, Concordia University-St. Paul, St. Paul, Minnesota

JOSE A. RAMIREZ – DEL TORO, MD, Fellow, Sports Medicine and Spinal Intervention, Mountainside Hospital, Montclair New Jersey

CARA CAMIOLO REDDY, MD, Assistant Professor, Department of Physical Medicine and Rehabilitation, University of Pittsburgh Medical Center, Pittsburgh, Pennsylvania

HUA MING SIOW, MBChB, MMed, FRCSEd, Fellow, Department of Orthopaedic Surgery, Children's Hospital of Philadelphia, Philadelphia, Pennsylvania; and Associate Consultant, Department of Orthopaedic Surgery, KK Women's and Children's Hospital, Singapore

AYNSLEY M. SMITH, RN, PhD, Sport Psychology Consultant and Research Director, Mayo Clinic Sports Medicine Center; Associate Professor, Department of Orthopedic Surgery and Physical Medicine and Rehabilitation, Mayo Medical School, Rochester, Minnesota

CHRISTOPHER J. STANDAERT, MD, Clinical Associate Professor, Departments of Rehabilitation Medicine, Orthopaedic and Sports Medicine, and Neurological Surgery, University of Washington, Seattle, Washington

ANDREW TUCKER, MD, Medical Director of Sports Medicine, Union Memorial Hospital, Baltimore, Maryland

JEFFREY M. VAUGHN, DO, Fellow, Division of Sports Medicine, Boston Children's Hospital, Boston, Massachusetts

BRANDEE L. WAITE, MD, Assistant Professor, Sports Medicine Fellowship Co-Director, University of California Davis Sports Medicine; Physical Medicine and Rehabilitation, University of California Davis School of Medicine, Sacramento, California

CONTENTS

> Childhood obesity is a key public health issue in the United States and around the globe in developed and developing countries. Obese children are at increased risk of acute medical illnesses and chronic diseases—in particular, osteoarthritis, diabetes mellitus, and cardiovascular disease, which can lead to poor quality of life; increased personal and financial burden to individuals, families, and society; and shortened lifespan. Physical inactivity and sedentary lifestyle are associated with being overweight in children and adults. Thus it is imperative to consider exercise and physical activity as a means to prevent and combat the childhood obesity epidemic. Familiarity with definitions of weight status in children and health outcomes like metabolic syndrome is crucial in understanding the literature on childhood obesity. Exercise and physical activity play a role in weight from the prenatal through adolescent time frame. A child's family and community impact access to adequate physical activity, and further study of these upstream issues is warranted. Recommended levels of physical activity for childhood obesity prevention are being developed.

> With the exception of Rhode Island, all states require high school athletes to undergo a preparticipation examination. These

examinations may vary from state to state, however. This article covers the basics of the history, physical examination, special tests, and issues surrounding clearance for various diagnoses.

In recent years there has been a significant increase in the number of youth participating in organized and competitive sports. Recent studies have supported the participation of preadolescent athletes in strength training to improve health and performance in sports. This article presents the most recent data available to help youth develop a safe and effective strength training program. Variables, such as the recommended rate of progression, the number of sets and repetitions an athlete should perform on each exercise, and how often an athlete needs to workout to avoid loss of strength achieved during a period of strength training are presented.

Approximately 2 million sports and recreation concussive injuries occur per year in the United States, which may be an underestimate because of inconsistent data reporting. The field of concussion management has evolved rapidly over the last 10 years, and with these advances comes new understanding of the significant symptomatic and cognitive impairments of concussion. These sequelae are more fully realized and may last longer than previously thought. Data have emerged regarding pathophysiology of concussion, risk factors, outcome, effects of repetitive injury, subtypes of concussive injury, and treatment protocols. This evidence calls for more conservative management of concussion, particularly in younger athletes, and demonstrates the short-comings of concussion guidelines.

The shoulder and elbow represent two of the most commonly injured joints in the adolescent population. Specific injuries vary by sport and can involve various structures, depending on the mechanism of injury. Unlike the adult shoulder, the immature skeletal structure of the adolescent athlete can lead to several unique injuries. By understanding the special demands placed on the immature shoulder, the sports physician can more effectively treat the resultant injury. This article reviews the diagnosis and management of unique injuries to the shoulder and elbow in the adolescent athlete.

CONTENTS

FORTHCOMING ISSUES

RECENT ISSUES

VISIT OUR WEB SITE

The Clinics are now available online!
Access your subscription at www.theclinics.com

ELSEVIER
SAUNDERS

Phys Med Rehabil Clin N Am
19 (2008) xiii–xiv

PHYSICAL MEDICINE
AND REHABILITATION
CLINICS OF
NORTH AMERICA

Foreword

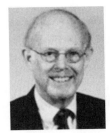

George H. Kraft, MD, MS
Consulting Editor

> The Battle of Waterloo was won on the playing fields of Eton.
>
> —*Attributed to the Duke of Wellington (1769–1852)*

I don't know if the Duke of Wellington ever actually said the quotation above, but it makes some sense. Athletic prowess obtained during the stage of physical growth and development would surely have been a powerful factor for victory in any nineteenth century land battle. Child and adolescent athletics may not have the same importance for national survival in today's computer era, but they are important for health and well being. And they can be fun. But they can also be dangerous: hence, this issue of *Clinics*.

It is a truism that a child is not just a miniature adult. During the period of human growth and development, the nonmature skeleton may be more prone to injury, and injuries may have long-term consequences. Sports medicine delivered to a child or adolescent athlete will be different from that delivered to a fully developed adult. Still, although intuitively known, this may not be fully appreciated. Even though a higher percentage of school-aged children than adults play sports (think of all of the soccer, T-ball and baseball, football, basketball, wrestling, and other sports children in primary and secondary grades play), the focus of most sports medicine is the adult athlete. But Guest Editor Dr. Brian Krabak and his talented coauthors have set out to change that. They have created an excellent and useful stand-alone book on management of injuries in the child and adolescent athlete.

1047-9651/08/$ - see front matter © 2008 Elsevier Inc. All rights reserved.
doi:10.1016/j.pmr.2008.01.003

pmr.theclinics.com

Dr. Krabak is likely no stranger to readers of the *Physical Medicine and Rehabilitation Clinics of North America*. He is well known as one of the co-authors of the *Physical Medicine and Rehabilitation Pocketpedia* [1]. His field of interest is sports medicine, and he is world-renowned as a physician for various world-wide extreme athletic events, such as the recent "4 Deserts" series of endurance races, which has earned him the title "Dr. Extreme," recently given to him by the *Seattle Times* [2].

Dr. Krabak understands the differences between adult sports injuries and those of skeletally immature athletes. In this issue of the *Clinics*, he and his colleagues discuss musculoskeletal injuries (shoulder, elbow, spine, pelvis, hip, knee, ankle, and foot), as well as head injury, strength training, and sport performance in this population. Finally, Dr. Krabak and his colleagues cover the preparticipatation physical examination, nutritional requirements for these student-athletes, and exercises to prevent childhood obesity. These are all important topics.

Although there are many books written for parents on their children's athletics (Amazon lists over 200), there are very few for physicians. Dr. Krabak and his colleagues have written a very useful guide for any physician seeing injured children in his or her practice. I am sure that the reader will find this issue both fascinating and useful.

George H. Kraft, MD, MS
*Alvord Professor of MS Research
Professor, Rehabilitation Medicine
Adjunct Professor, Neurology
University of Washington
Box 356490
1959 NE Pacific Street
Seattle, WA 98195-6490, USA*

E-mail address: ghkraft@u.washington.edu

References

[1] Choi H, Sugar R, Fish D, et al. Physical Medicine & Rehabilitation Pocketpedia. Philadelphia: Lippincott Williams & Wilkins; 2003.
[2] Seven R. "Dr. Extreme studies athletes who push through pain." *Seattle Times*, Nov 12, 2007.

ELSEVIER
SAUNDERS

Phys Med Rehabil Clin N Am
19 (2008) xv–xvi

PHYSICAL MEDICINE
AND REHABILITATION
CLINICS OF
NORTH AMERICA

Preface

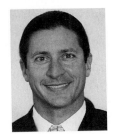

Brian J. Krabak, MD, MBA
Guest Editor

We are living in a time of contradiction in regards to the health and activity of children and adolescents. On the one hand, we are faced with rampant and worsening childhood obesity that is multifactorial in nature. Contributing causes include decreased physical activity, poor parental role models, poor eating habits, and dwindling support for physical fitness programs in the school systems. On the other hand, physically fit children are now competing in multiple sports throughout the year without periods of rest. Competitive sports have become "too competitive," as children attempt to emulate professional athletes and respond to the pressure of parents, coaches, and their peers. Such continuous training and pressure can potentially lead to an increase in injuries and loss of perspective for the benefits of exercise.

The Child and Adolescent Athlete provides a comprehensive, multidisciplinary, state-of-the art review focusing on the athlete as a whole. This issue of *Clinics* will explore the impact of inactivity and excessive activity on the musculoskeletal, neurologic, psychologic, and nutritional aspects of the child and adolescent athlete. By understanding the spectrum of disorders relating to obesity and sport-specific activities, the physician will be able to assist the athlete and their family throughout the treatment process, and

1047-9651/08/$ - see front matter © 2008 Elsevier Inc. All rights reserved.
doi:10.1016/j.pmr.2008.01.001

pmr.theclinics.com

hopefully establish a foundation of respect toward activity and fitness for the rest of the child's life.

Brian J. Krabak, MD, MBA
Clinical Associate Professor
University of Washington Sports and Spine Rehabilitation
Children's Hospital and Regional Medical Center
Departments of Rehabilitation, Orthopaedics and Sports Medicine
Team Consultant, University of Washington
1959 NE Pacific Street, Box 356490
Seattle, Washington 98195

E-mail address: bkrabak@u.washington.edu

ELSEVIER
SAUNDERS

Phys Med Rehabil Clin N Am
19 (2008) 205–216

PHYSICAL MEDICINE
AND REHABILITATION
CLINICS OF
NORTH AMERICA

Exercise for Preventing Childhood Obesity

Sheila A. Dugan, MD[a,b,*]

[a]*Department of PM&R, University PM&R, Rush Medical College, 1725 West Harrison
Street, Suite 970, Chicago, IL 60612, USA*
[b]*Department of Preventive Medicine, University PM&R, Rush Medical College,
1700 West Van Buren Street, Suite 470, Chicago, IL 60612, USA*

Childhood obesity is a key public health issue in the United States and has been referred to as a global epidemic and public health crisis [1–3]. Obese children are at increased risk of acute medical illnesses, including asthma and high blood pressure, and chronic diseases—in particular, osteoarthritis, diabetes mellitus, and cardiovascular disease [4]. Physical inactivity and sedentary lifestyle are associated with being overweight in children and adults. Thus it is imperative to consider exercise and physical activity as a means to prevent and combat the childhood obesity epidemic.

Definitions

Obesity and overweight are defined in terms of body mass index (BMI). BMI is used to define categories of weight status as it relates to health. BMI is a value derived by using height and weight measurements (weight in kg/height in m^2) that gives a general indication of whether weight falls within a healthy range. For adults, BMI strongly correlates with total body fat content as it describes weight relative to height. For children, BMI-for-age is an important concept as children's body fat changes over the years as they grow (Fig. 1). In addition, boys and girls differ in body fatness as they mature. The National Institutes of Health and Centers for Disease Control and Prevention use the terms *underweight, normal weight, overweight,* and *obese* in adults according to cut-points in BMI and related to BMI-for-age in children, rather than the traditional height/weight charts (Table 1) [5]. For children, underweight is defined as BMI at or below 5th

---

* University PM&R, Rush Medical College, 1725 West Harrison Street, Suite 970, Chicago, IL 60612.
E-mail address: sheila_dugan@rush.edu

1047-9651/08/$ - see front matter © 2008 Elsevier Inc. All rights reserved.
doi:10.1016/j.pmr.2007.11.001
pmr.theclinics.com

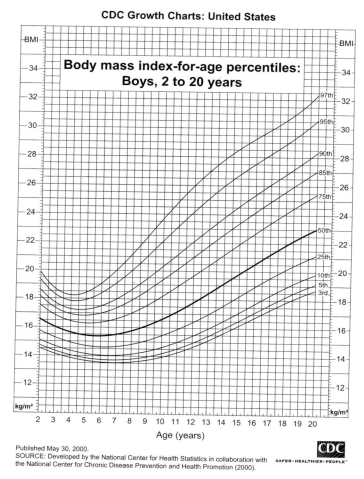

Published May 30, 2000.
SOURCE: Developed by the National Center for Health Statistics in collaboration with SAFER·HEALTHIER·PEOPLE™
the National Center for Chronic Disease Prevention and Health Promotion (2000).

Fig. 1. BMI-for-age for boys 2–20 years old. (*Reprinted from* the National Center for Health Statistics in collaboration with the National Center for Chronic Disease Prevention and Health Promotion (200), May 30, 2000, Centers for Disease Control and Prevention. http://www.cdc.gov/nchs/about/major/nhanes/growthcharts/clinical_charts.htm.)

percentile of the sex-specific BMI-for-age growth chart. At risk for overweight is defined as BMI at or above 85th percentile of the sex-specific BMI-for-age growth chart. Overweight is defined as BMI at or above 95th percentile of the sex-specific BMI-for-age growth chart (Fig. 2). Across many studies, childhood obesity was defined as BMI at or above 85th percentile for age and sex.

A recent meta-analysis reported rising numbers of overweight and obese adults and overweight children over the last four decades [6]. A large epidemiologic study, part of the National Health and Nutrition Examination Survey (NHANES), demonstrated that the numbers of overweight children

Table 1
Weight status categories for percentile range of BMI-for-age for individuals 2–20 years of age

Weight status category	Percentile range
Underweight	Less than the 5th percentile
Healthy weight	5th to less than the 85th percentile
At risk of overweight	85th to less than the 95th percentile
Overweight	Equal to or greater than the 95th percentile

Adapted from the Centers for Disease Control and Prevention, Division of Nutrition, Physical Activity and Obesity in collaboration with the National Center for Chronic Disease Prevention and Health Promotion. CDC.gov, May 2007. http://www.cdc.gov/nccdphp/dnpa/bmi/childrens_BMI/about_childrens_BMI.htm.

are on the rise [7]. NHANES measured height and weight in more than 4000 adults and 4000 children from 1999 to 2000 and then again from 2001 to 2002. Among children 6 through 19 years of age from 1999 to 2002, 31% were at risk for overweight or overweight and 16% were overweight. Both the meta-analysis and NHANES results indicate continuing disparities in the burden of overweight and obesity by sex and between racial/ethnic groups and related to socioeconomic status.

The metabolic syndrome is a cluster of conditions that often occur together, including obesity, high blood pressure, glucose intolerance, and dyslipidemia [8]. These clinical measures assess the cardiovascular disease risk profile of the individual. Metabolic syndrome is a clinical outcome of being overweight or obese that goes beyond measuring BMI only. Metabolic syndrome allows for assessment of the negative health consequences of being overweight and obese. Components of the metabolic syndrome have been studied in children and adolescents related to birth weight, indicating that the intrauterine environment already plays a role in childhood weight status and health outcomes [9,10].

Weight status is highly dependent on energy consumed versus energy burned or expended. Physical activity is one of the modifiable components of total energy expenditure, which also includes gender, age, current body weight, basal metabolic rate and, in childhood, the energy cost of growth [11]. The energy cost of growth has two components: (1) the energy needed to synthesize growing tissues and (2) the energy deposited in those tissues. The energy cost of growth is about 35% of total energy requirement during the first 3 months of age, falls rapidly to about 5% at 12 months and about 3% in the second year, remains at 1% to 2% until mid-adolescence, and is negligible in the late teens.

Physical activity not only plays a significant role in expending energy, but also directly impacts physiologic parameters related to weight gain, mainly via fat and glucose metabolism [12]. Skeletal muscle plays a major role in the daily fat oxidation in the body. Physical activity controls fat mass by increasing the amount of fat oxidized at the skeletal muscle. Skeletal muscle also serves as an active reservoir of glucose, and regular physical activity promotes insulin sensitivity and glucose homeostasis independently of its

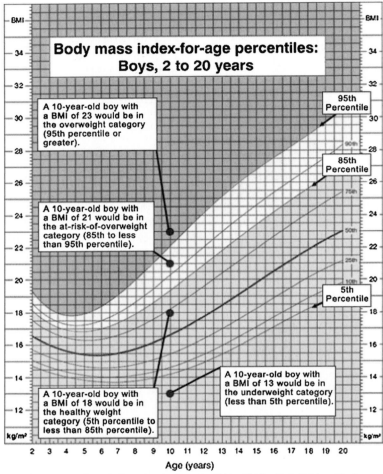

Source: Developed by the Centers for Disease Control and Prevention, Division of Nutrition, Physical Activity and Obesity in collaboration with the National Center for Chronic Disease Prevention and Health Promotion. CDC.gov, May 2007.

Fig. 2. BMI-for-age chart with examples of how some sample BMI numbers would be interpreted for a 10-year-old boy. (*Reprinted from* the Centers for Disease Control and Prevention, Division of Nutrition, Physical Activity and Obesity in collaboration with the National Center for Chronic Disease Prevention and Health Promotion. CDC.gov, May 2007. http://www.cdc. gov/nccdphp/dnpa/bmi/childrens_BMI/about_childrens_BMI.htm.)

effect on body fat. Exercise also plays a direct role in improving heath outcomes, such as reducing one's risk of cardiovascular disease.

Prenatal factors

Exercise in pregnancy has been shown to play an important role in preventing chronic health conditions in women [13]. Of interest to this review, exercise in pregnancy was also shown to be beneficial to the growing fetus. Although it is known that women with diabetes mellitus, gestational diabetes mellitus (GDM), or obesity tend to have larger babies [14], the benefits of exercise to normalize infant birth weight are not as widely considered. Women who are the most physically active have the lowest prevalence of GDM, and prevention of GDM may decrease the incidence of obesity and type 2 diabetes in both mother and offspring [15].

Macrosomia leads not only to increase cesarean section and shoulder dystocia rate [14], but also to negative health outcomes to the child. A longitudinal cohort study in the United States compared children 6 to 11 years old who were large-for-gestational-age versus appropriate-for-gestational-age at birth [9]. Clinical outcomes measured in the study included the metabolic syndrome—obesity (BMI $\geq$ 85th percentile for age), hypertension, dyslipidemia, and glucose intolerance. They found that children exposed to maternal obesity were at increased risk of developing metabolic syndrome, which suggests that obese mothers who do not fulfill the clinical criteria for GDM may still have metabolic factors that affect fetal growth and postnatal outcomes. A retrospective chart review of a multi-ethnic, low-income cohort of children demonstrated that maternal obesity in early pregnancy more than doubled the risk of obesity at 2 to 4 years of age [16]. The researcher concluded that in developing strategies to prevent obesity in preschoolers, special attention should be given to newborns with obese mothers. Chinese researchers evaluated the relationship between birth weight and cardiovascular disease risk factors in children and adolescents in more than 80,000 children [10]. High birth weight was correlated with childhood obesity and diabetes. Low birth weight was also associated with childhood diabetes. The researchers concluded that a different relationship existed between the high- and low-birth weight children and the development of obesity, hypertension, and diabetes in childhood. These studies strongly suggest that the long-term health trajectory of the individual vis-à-vis obesity is partially impacted by the fetal environment.

Antepartum issues: infancy and preschool years

Physical activity has not been studied in early infancy as a means of preventing childhood obesity. Rather, nutrition—breast-feeding in particular—has been studied most related to infant weight. For instance, one study correlated rapid infant weight gain from birth to 6 months with childhood overweight at 4 years of age [17]. There is a natural phenomenon of increasing adiposity during the first year of life, then a decrease until a second rise in adiposity at about 5 to 6 years old. The term *adiposity rebound* has been given to the phenomenon of this second increase in adiposity (Fig. 3) [18]. Studies have shown a relationship between the age at adiposity rebound and final adult adiposity. An early rebound (before 5.5 years of age) was followed by a significantly higher adiposity level than a later rebound (after

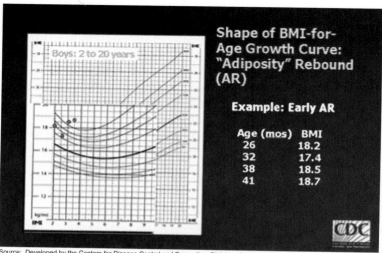

Fig. 3. BMI-for-age chart with example of adiposity rebound. (Reprinted from the Centers for
Disease Control and Prevention, Division of Nutrition, Physical Activity and Obesity in collaboration with the National Center for Chronic Disease Prevention and Health Promotion.
CDC.gov, May 2007. http://www.cdc.gov/nccdphp/dnpa/growthcharts/training/modules/
module1/text/page4btext.htm.)

7 years of age) in one study [19], whereas a second study showed that
adiposity rebound before ages 4 to 6 was associated with obesity in adulthood [20]. The preschool years are thought to be a critical period for obesity
prevention as indicated by the association of the adiposity rebound and obesity in later years; however, there is limited research addressing the role of
exercise and physical activity in obesity prevention in preschool aged
children [21].

A recent meta-analysis found only 7 studies of physical activity interventions in preschool-age children (2–6 years old) for obesity prevention and
obesity treatment [22]. All of the studies included multiple components,
not just physical activity interventions, but also diet and family lifestyle
modification. Four of the 7 studies (2 intervention, 2 prevention) documented significant reductions in weight status or body fat. Another meta-
analysis identified 11 studies of children 0 to 5 years of age that targeted
overweight with multimodal strategies related to physical activity, sedentary
behavior, and diet [23]. All studies had success in changing at least one negative health behavior related to weight management, and the authors concluded that parents are receptive to and capable of some behavioral
changes that may promote healthy weight in their young children. One
methodological issue in this age group that may limit research is accurate
measurement of physical activity. Parental report of outdoor playtime in
preschool-age children correlated highly with objective measurement with

accelerometers, providing evidence that parental survey may be a worthwhile method for future studies in this age group [24].

School-age children

There is a large literature addressing obesity prevention and treatment in school-age children. A recent review was undertaken to synthesize these studies to develop best practice recommendations [21]. This included a critical appraisal of the myriad studies for the prevention and treatment of childhood obesity (and associated chronic diseases) that are published. Researchers found that a multifaceted approach to obesity prevention was crucial, not only on the individual level (eg, promoting healthy food choices and increased exercise), but also on the societal level (eg, investing in safe parks and gymnasiums). School and the community emerged as the best settings for implementation of multidimensional strategies. Children spend considerable time in school, and schools offer the opportunity to interface with at-risk children [25].

In regards to physical activity as the primary intervention in obesity treatment, a meta-analysis reviewed 8 studies of otherwise healthy 4- to 17-year-olds enrolled in exercise interventions that included walking, jogging, cycle aerometry, high-repetition resistance exercise, and combinations of at least 8-week duration with at least six subjects per group [26]. They included studies that had pre- and posttest measures of body composition. They concluded that exercise interventions were effective in reducing percentage body fat in obese children and adolescents. Another review with similar but slightly different inclusion criteria (eg, exercise intervention for at least 3 weeks and 5- to 17-year-old children) analyzed 30 studies of exercise intervention to treat obesity in childhood [27]. Fixed-effects modeling combining the results of the 30 studies demonstrated statistically significant in selected body composition variables in the exercise intervention group. Stepwise linear regression suggested that initial body fat levels (or body mass), type of treatment intervention, exercise intensity, and exercise mode accounted for most of the variance associated with changes in body composition after training. Germane to the present article, exercise interventions for preventing childhood obesity have been studied [28–31]. There was a wide range of physical activity measurements and varying exercise regiments used across the studies, similar to the range seen in exercise studies to treat obesity in childhood.

Family issues

There is evidence that targeting parental behaviors may be more effective than interventions directed solely toward children to combat childhood obesity [32]. Although there is a significant literature on parental inputs on nutritional issues related to offspring obesity, the literature on parental physical activity related to offspring obesity is not as extensive. Researchers in Spain evaluated 14 interventional studies and concluded that nutritional education and promotion of physical activity, together with behavior modifications, decrease in sedentary activities, and the collaboration of the family, could be the determining factors in the prevention of childhood obesity [33]. It is crucial to consider interventions or programs that modify the environment that a child is exposed to during early development to have a lasting effect on weight.

Community issues

Although the majority of this article thus far has reviewed exercise interventions to individuals, described as downstream intervention, upstream investment and intervention for community programs and facilities that make physical activity accessible and fun for children are paramount. Researchers have concluded that there is an opportunity to develop more upstream and population-focused interventions and programs to balance and extend the current emphasis on individual-based programs that dominates the literature [21]. They also noted limited study of the downstream (individual) or upstream (family or community) factors that may contribute to obesity in special populations, such as immigrants, new to developed countries, who may be more vulnerable to the obesogenic environment. It is not clear how large a role a sedentary lifestyle plays in obesogeneity for each special population; however, it is clear that lack of exercise and reduced physical activity in this country's 9.4 million children with disabilities and special health care needs put them at increased risk of obesity and cardiovascular disease [34]. Accessible playgrounds, pools, and gymnasiums would facilitate increased physical activity for all children, but require visions of inclusion and financial resources. In a national sample of women with young children living in low-income urban environments, obesity was more prevalent among those who perceived their neighborhoods to be unsafe [35]. Safety concerns limited physical activity and outdoor playtime.

Specific physical activity recommendations for obesity prevention in childhood

There are several studies that analyzed step counts by pedometer-assessed steps per day (SPD) and developed specific recommendations on cut-points for obesity prevention. Step counts in almost 2000 children 6 to 12 years old from the United States, Australia, and Sweden with healthy body composition (based on normal range BMI-for-age) were analyzed by American researchers [36]. Their recommended cut-points for SPD for healthy body composition were 12,000 SPD for girls and 15,000 SPD for boys. More recent recommendations based on a more specific measure of healthy body composition of almost 1000 New Zealander, European, Polynesian, and Asian children 5 to 12 years old and using body fat percent measured with hand-to-foot bioelectrical impedance analysis increased the cut-points by 1000 steps [37]. They recommended 13,000 SPD for girls and 16,000 SPD for boys for healthy body composition. Of note, a recent study of over 200 British primary school children found that the majority of children did not meet the health-related BMI-for-age–determined cut-points [38]. They also found a statistically significant difference in physical activity during week-days compared with weekends, with fewer steps taken on weekends. Overall, boys were more active than girls and they attained statistically significantly higher mean SPD than girls. Forty-four seventh-grade girls and boys in the United States were studied over 2 weeks of consistent pedometer wear. The total sample mean was 11,392 SPD, SD = 4112; the mean for boys was 12,490 SPD, SD = 3910, versus the mean for girls, which was 10,557 SPD [39]. They noted that students involved in after-school activities had higher step counts and that after-school activities and physical education class combined to account for an average of 65% of the step count.

In keeping with adult public health recommendations of exercise for healthy body composition, one can consider counseling children based on minutes of moderate-intensity cardiovascular exercise or aerobic physical activity. The recently updated joint American College of Sports Medicine and American Heart Association recommendations were for 30 minutes of moderate-intensity exercise five times per week or 20 minutes of vigorous exercise three times per week for health promotion for adults 18 to 65 years of age [40]. In a study of adults who wore both accelerometer and pedom-eter, researchers were able to identify a value of pedometer-SPD that closely corresponded with the recommended 30 min/day of moderate ambulatory activity [41]. They concluded that approximately 33 min/day of moderate activity per accelerometer corresponded with 8000 pedometer-SPD. They noted that further studies with distinct populations (eg, children and adoles-cents) were warranted to confirm a recommended number of SPD associ-ated with the duration and intensity of public health-recommended ambulatory activity.

Interestingly, a meta-analysis of evidence-based physical activity inter-vention studies for school-age youths recommended that they partake daily in 60 minutes or more of moderate to vigorous physical activity that is de-velopmentally appropriate and enjoyable and involves a variety of activities to garner health benefits, one of which was weight management [42]. Using the adult estimates of accelerometer versus pedometer measures, 60 minutes of moderate exercise would correlate with 15,000 to 16,000 SPD. This is in line with the SPD recommended for boys based on body fat percent and BMI-for-age calculations as listed above but slightly higher than SPD rec-ommended for girls. In addition, the recommended dosing for health pro-motion for adults is 5 days per week rather than daily, as recommended by these researchers.

Summary

Childhood obesity is an important public health problem throughout the world. Although this article focuses on the role of exercise and physical activity in the prevention of childhood obesity, one must address prevention from many angles, including nutrition and lifestyle. Using BMI for identifying overweight and at-risk of overweight children is key as it serves as an indicator of body fatness. In children as well as adults, elevated BMI is associated with increased cardiovascular disease health risk, both short and long term. Identification of critical periods for the development of obesity (such as the timing of the adiposity rebound) can help with targeting prevention strategies. Moderate to vigorous physical activity is needed to convey health benefits in children and adults. To improve compliance, activity should be developmentally appropriate and enjoyable and involve a variety of activities.

References

[1] Ebbeling CB, Rawlak DB, Ludwig DS. Childhood obesity: public-health crisis, common sense cure. Lancet 2002;360:473–82.
[2] Lobstein T, Baur L, Uauy R. Obesity in children and young people: a crisis in public health. Obes Rev 2004;5(Suppl 1):4–85.
[3] WHO. Obesity, preventing and managing the global epidemic. Report of a WHO Consultation. Geneva (Switzerland): World Health Organization; June 3–5, 2000.
[4] Cymet TC. Childhood obesity: normal variant or serious illness? Compr Ther 2006;32(3): 147–9.
[5] Centers for Disease Control and Prevention, Division of Nutrition, Physical Activity and Obesity in collaboration with the National Center for Chronic Disease Prevention and Health Promotion. CDC.gov. Accessed May 2007.
[6] Wang Y, Beydoun MA. The obesity epidemic in the united states—gender, age, socioeconomic, racial/ethnic, and geographic characteristics: a systematic review and meta-regression analysis. Epidemiol Rev 2007;29(1):6–28.
[7] Hedley AA, Ogden CL, Johnson CL, et al. Prevalence of overweight and obesity among US children, adolescents, and adults, 1999–2002. JAMA 2004;291:2847–50.
[8] Grundy SM, Brewer HB, Cleeman JI, et al. Definition of metabolic syndrome: report of the National Heart, Lung, and Blood Institute/American Heart Association conference on scientific issues related to definition. Circulation 2004;109:433–8.
[9] Boney CM, Verma A, Tucker R, et al. Metabolic syndrome in childhood: association with birth weight, maternal obesity, and gestational diabetes mellitus. Pediatrics 2005;115(3): e290–6.
[10] Wei JN, Li HY, Sung FC, et al. Birth weight correlates differently with cardiovascular risk factors in youth. Obesity (Silver Spring) 2007;15:1609–16.
[11] WHO. Energy and protein requirements: report of a joint FAO/WHO/UNU expert consultation. Geneva (Switzerland): WHO; Technical Report Series No. 724; 1985.
[12] Maffeis C, Castellani M. Physical activity: an effective way to control weight in children? Nutr Metab Cardiovasc Dis 2007;17(5):394–408.
[13] Pivarnik JM, Chambliss HO, Clapp JF, et al. Impact of physical activity during pregnancy and postpartum on chronic disease risk. Special Communications. Med Sci Sports Exerc 2006;38(5):989–1006.

[14] Chatfield J. ACOG issues guidelines on fetal macrosomia. American College of Obstetrics and Gynecology. Am Fam Physician 2001;64(1):169–70.

[15] Weissgerber TL, Wolfe LA, Davies GA, et al. Exercise in the prevention and treatment of maternal-fetal disease: a review of the literature. Appl Physiol Nutr Metab 2006;31(6): 661–74.

[16] Whitaker RC. Predicting preschooler obesity at birth: the role of maternal obesity in early pregnancy. Pediatrics 2004;114(1):e29–36.

[17] Dennison BA, Edmunds LS, Stratton HH, et al. Rapid infant weight gain predicts childhood overweight. Obesity (Silver Spring) 2006;14:491–9.

[18] Whitaker RC, Wright JA, Pepe MS, et al. Predicting obesity in young adulthood from childhood and parental obesity. N Engl J Med 1997;37(13):869–73.

[19] Rolland-Cachera MF, Deheeger M, Maillot M, et al. Early adiposity rebound: causes, and consequences for obesity in children and adults. Int J Obes (Lond) 2006;30(Suppl):S11–7.

[20] Whitaker RC, Pepe MS, Wright JA, et al. Early adiposity rebound and the risk of adult obesity. Pediatrics 1998;101(3):E5, Abstract.

[21] Flynn MA, McNeil DA, Maloff B, et al. Reducing obesity and related chronic disease risk in children and youth: a synthesis of evidence with 'best practice' recommendations. Obes Rev 2006;7(Suppl 1):7–66.

[22] Bluford DAA, Sherry B, Scanlon KS. Interventions to prevent or treat obesity in preschool children: a review of evaluated programs. Obesity (Silver Spring) 2007;15:1356–72.

[23] Campbell KJ, Hesketh KD. Strategies which aim to positively impact on weight, physical activity, diet and sedentary behaviours in children from zero to five years. A systematic review of the literature. Obes Rev 2007;8(4):327–38.

[24] Burdette HL, Whitaker RC, Daniels SR. Parental report of outdoor playtime as a measure of physical activity in preschool-aged children. Arch Pediatr Adolesc Med 2004;158(4):353–7.

[25] WHO. Expert Committee on Comprehensive School Health Education and Promotion. Promoting Health Through Schools. Geneva (Switzerland): World Health Organization; 1997.

[26] Andreacci JL, LeMura LM, Stoddard NM, et al. Follow up exercise studies in paediatric obesity: implications for long term effectiveness. Br J Sports Med 2003;37(5):425–9.

[27] LeMura LM, Maziekas MT. Factors that alter body fat, body mass and fat free mass in pediatric obesity. Med Sci Sports Exerc 2002;34(3):487–96.

[28] Campbell K, Waters E, O'Meara S, et al. Interventions for preventing obesity in children. The Cochrane Collaboration. Available at: http://80-gateway1.ovid.com.ezproxy.lib. ucalgary.ca:2048/ovidweb.cgi. Accessed February 27, 2002.

[29] Hardeman W, Griffin S, Johnston M, et al. Interventions to prevent weight gain: a systematic review of psychological models and behaviour change methods. Int J Obes Relat Metab Disord 2000;24:131–43.

[30] Jerum A, Melnyk BM. Effectiveness of interventions to prevent obesity and obesity related complications in children and adolescents. Pediatr Nurs 2001;27:606–10.

[31] Resnicow K. School-based obesity prevention: population versus high-risk interventions. Ann N Y Acad Sci 1993;699:154–66.

[32] Agras WS, Mascola AJ. Risk factors for childhood overweight. Curr Opin Pediatr 2005; 17(5):648–52.

[33] Bautista-Castano I, Doreste J, Serra-Majem L. Effectiveness of interventions in the prevention of childhood obesity. Eur J Epidemiol 2004;19(7):617–22.

[34] Minihan PM, Fitch SM, Must A. What does the epidemic of childhood obesity mean for children with special health care needs? J Law Med Ethics 2007;35(1):61–77.

[35] Burdette HL, Wadden TA, Whitaker RC. Neighborhood safety, collective efficacy, and obesity in women with young children. Obesity (Silver Spring) 2006;14(3):518–25.

[36] Tudor-Locke C, Pangrazi RP, Corbin CB, et al. BMI-referenced standards for recommended pedometer-determined steps/day in children. Prev Med 2004;38:857–64.

[37] Duncan JS, Schofield G, Duncan EK. Step count recommendations for children based on body fat. Prev Med 2007;44(1):42–4.

[38] Duncan MJ, Al-Nakeeb Y, Woodfield L, et al. Pedometer determined physical activity levels in primary school children from central England. Prev Med 2007;44(5):416–20.
[39] Flohr JA, Todd MK, Tudor-Locke C. Pedometer-assessed physical activity in young adolescents. Res Q Exerc Sport 2006;77(3):309–15.
[40] Haskell WJ, Lee IM, Pate RR, et al. Physical activity and public health: updated recommendation for adults from the American College of Sports Medicine and the American Heart Association. Med Sci Sports Exerc 2007;39(8):1423–34.
[41] Tudor-Locke C, Ainsworth BE, Thompson RW, et al. Comparison of pedometer and accelerometer of free living physical activity. Med Sci Sports Exerc 2002;34(12):2045–51.
[42] Strong WB, Malina RM, Blimkie CJ, et al. Evidence based physical activity for school-age youth. J Pediatr 2005;146(6):732–7.

ELSEVIER
SAUNDERS

Phys Med Rehabil Clin N Am
19 (2008) 217–234

PHYSICAL MEDICINE
AND REHABILITATION
CLINICS OF
NORTH AMERICA

Role of the Adolescent Preparticipation Physical Examination

Andrew Tucker, MD[a],*, Matthew Grady, MD, FAAP[b]

[a]Union Memorial Hospital, 1407 York Road, Suite 100 A, Lutherville, MD 21093, USA
[b]Department of Orthopedics, Children's Hospital of Philadelphia, 34th and Civic Center
Boulevard, Second Floor, Wood Building, Philadelphia, PA 19104, USA

Each year over 7 million high school students participate in school-sponsored sports programs [1]. With the exception of Rhode Island, all states require a high school athlete to undergo a preparticipation examination (PPE); however, there is no uniform national standard regarding this common evaluation. In addition, states vary greatly as to who is allowed to perform the PPE. A few states allow clinicians other than physicians, including nurse practitioners, chiropractors, and physician assistants, to complete the examination and necessary paperwork.

The primary goal of the PPE is to make sports participation as safe as possible. The PPE attempts to identify any life-threatening (eg, cardiovascular defects) or potentially disabling conditions (eg, cervical stenosis) that may place a young athlete at risk on the playing field. Second, it aims to identify any orthopedic conditions that may predispose to injury (eg, shoulder instability) or medical conditions that may be worsened by sports participation (eg, exercise-induced asthma). A third major objective of the PPE is to fulfill state and local legal requirements for scholastic sports participation.

Several secondary objectives may be attained, depending on the specific goals and available resources of the medical staff, school, or community. These potential secondary goals include assessment of general health, fitness and performance assessment (eg, body composition, flexibility), and counseling on health-related matters. Studies indicate that a large number of adolescents use the PPE as their yearly health maintenance examination [2]. Therefore some clinicians advocate that the PPE serve other purposes including screening for high-risk behaviors, violence and safety issues,

* Corresponding author.
E-mail address: andrew.tucker@medstar.net (A. Tucker).

1047-9651/08/$ - see front matter © 2008 Elsevier Inc. All rights reserved.
doi:10.1016/j.pmr.2007.12.004

pmr.theclinics.com

tobacco/drug and alcohol use, sexuality, and emotional issues. Adolescent screening questionnaires, available from the American Medical Association at www.ama-assn.org/ama/pub/category/1980.html, may be used to help identify issues requiring further follow-up. Finally, simply notifying the parent(s) of the limitations of a screening PPE may encourage future follow-up care with the primary care physician.

Timing and location

The timing, location, and skill sets of the examiner(s) all impact the effectiveness of the PPE. Ideally, the examination should be done at least 4 to 6 weeks before the start of the sports season to allow time to address and correct any identified problems. The PPE typically is performed in one of two settings: an office-based examination by a primary care physician, or a mass screening station examination using multiple examiners. Each method has its own strengths and weakness, and it is important for examining physicians to anticipate the potential disadvantages of the method used (Table 1) [3]. With the athlete and/or parents' permission, anticipated medical problems and treatment plans should be discussed with sideline medical personnel, including coaches and athletic trainers.

The history

The most sensitive part of the evaluation is a thorough history. The history alone identifies approximately 75% of problems that may affect participation [4,5]. Several medical organizations (American Academy of

Table 1
Advantages and disadvantages of the office-based and station screening preparticipation examination

	Advantages	Disadvantages
Office-based	Established doctor–patient relationship	Variability of sports medicine interest and knowledge
	Follow-up care	Limited communication with team staff
	Private setting	Limited access
	Personal health counseling	Cost
	Communication with parents	
Station-based	Can use multiple specialized personal	Incomplete past medical history
	Time-efficient	No prior physician–patient relationship
	Cost-efficient	Lack of privacy
	School-based station examination can include coaches and athletic trainers.	Lack of continuity/follow-up issues
	Communication with school	Communication with parents

Pediatrics [AAP], American Academy of Family Physicians, AMSSM, AOSSM and AOASM) have published a monograph on the PPE (available at http://www.aap.org/bookstore/), which includes the medical history that is most pertinent to the young athlete. Previous studies have shown that an adolescent's recall about his or her past medical history is often incomplete [5]. Ideally, these forms should be completed by the parent first and then by the student athlete to respect privacy and obtain an accurate history (Fig. 1).

The past medical history should focus on past surgeries and major illnesses or chronic medical conditions that may be worsened by training and competition. Questions regarding previous illness or conditions should focus on hospitalizations or emergency room visits, adequacy of control of symptoms, and any current functional deficits. Athletes who have well-managed medical conditions, such as diabetes, asthma, and seizure, can participate in sports safely. The AAP has published extensive guidelines regarding medical conditions and sports participation. Table 2 highlights these guidelines, as does the section on medical clearance later in this article.

Medications/allergies

All medications, including over-the-counter medicines and nutritional supplements, should be reviewed. The examining physician should be aware of common medication complications in athletes who train at high levels, especially under severe environmental conditions. Stimulants, such as ephedra and anticholinergic medicines have been associated with significant heat illness. Methylxanthines, macrolide antibiotics, decongestants, and beta-agonists have been linked to arrhythmias. Fluoroquinolones, while not recommended for skeletally immature individuals, have been associated with tendon degeneration and Achilles tendon rupture and should not be used in athletes [6]. Questions regarding supplement use and anabolic steroids are likewise important. Current supplement trends include energy drinks and creatine. Creatine is used commonly by athletes of all ages primarily in strength and power sports, and its safety in young athletes has not been established. Energy drinks may contain large amounts of caffeine and other products such as ginseng, guarana, and taurine, to enhance the stimulant effect. Finally, certain classes of therapeutic drugs including diuretics, beta agonists, and stimulants, including attention-deficit hyperactive drugs are banned at the college and international level. A prescription is not sufficient to allow use, but approval for some medications may be granted after letters of medical necessity. Complete lists from the National Collegiate Athletic Association (NCAA) (http://www1.ncaa.org/membership/ed_outreach/health-safety/drug_testing/banned_drug_classes.pdf) and the world antidoping agency (http://www.wada-ama.org/en/prohibitedlist.ch2) are available on-line. Team physicians who care for athletes who will be drug tested are advised to be familiar with the relevant guidelines.

Preparticipation Physical Evaluation

HISTORY FORM

DATE OF EXAM_____

Name_____ Sex_____ Age_____ Date of birth_____

Grade____ School _____ Sport(s)_____

Address_____ Phone_____

Personal physician_____

In case of emergency, contact

Name _____ Relationship _____ Phone (H) _____ (W)_____

Explain "Yes" answers below.
Circle questions you don't know the answers to.

	Yes	No
1. Has a doctor ever denied or restricted your participation in sports for any reason?	☐	☐
2. Do you have an ongoing medical condition (like diabetes or asthma)?	☐	☐
3. Are you currently taking any prescription or nonprescription (over-the-counter) medicines or pills?	☐	☐
4. Do you have allergies to medicines, pollens, foods, or stinging insects?	☐	☐
5. Have you ever passed out or nearly passed out DURING exercise?	☐	☐
6. Have you ever passed out or nearly passed out AFTER exercise?	☐	☐
7. Have you ever had discomfort, pain, or pressure in your chest during exercise?	☐	☐
8. Does your heart race or skip beats during exercise?	☐	☐
9. Has a doctor ever told you that you have (check all that apply):		
☐ High blood pressure ☐ A heart murmur		
☐ High cholesterol ☐ A heart infection		
10. Has a doctor ever ordered a test for your heart? (for example, ECG, echocardiogram)	☐	☐
11. Has anyone in your family died for no apparent reason?	☐	☐
12. Does anyone in your family have a heart problem?	☐	☐
13. Has any family member or relative died of heart problems or of sudden death before age 50?	☐	☐
14. Does anyone in your family have Marfan syndrome?	☐	☐
15. Have you ever spent the night in a hospital?	☐	☐
16. Have you ever had surgery?	☐	☐
17. Have you ever had an injury, like a sprain, muscle or ligament tear or tendinitis, that caused you to miss a practice or game? If yes, circle affected area below:	☐	☐
18. Have you had any broken or fractured bones, or dislocated joints? If yes, circle below:	☐	☐
19. Have you had a bone or joint injury that required x-rays, MRI, CT, surgery, injections, rehabilitation, physical therapy, a brace, a cast, or crutches? If yes, circle below:	☐	☐

Head	Neck	Shoulder	Upper arm	Elbow	Forearm	Hand/ fingers	Chest
Upper back	Lower back	Hip	Thigh	Knee	Calf/shin	Ankle	Foot/toes

	Yes	No
20. Have you ever had a stress fracture?	☐	☐
21. Have you been told that you have or have you had an x-ray for atlantoaxial (neck) instability?	☐	☐
22. Do you regularly use a brace or assistive device?	☐	☐
23. Has a doctor ever told you that you have asthma or allergies?	☐	☐

	Yes	No
24. Do you cough, wheeze, or have difficulty breathing during or after exercise?	☐	☐
25. Is there anyone in your family who has asthma?	☐	☐
26. Have you ever used an inhaler or taken asthma medicine?	☐	☐
27. Were you born without or are you missing a kidney, an eye, a testicle, or any other organ?	☐	☐
28. Have you had infectious mononucleosis (mono) within the last month?	☐	☐
29. Do you have any rashes, pressure sores, or other skin problems?	☐	☐
30. Have you had a herpes skin infection?	☐	☐
31. Have you ever had a head injury or concussion?	☐	☐
32. Have you been hit in the head and been confused or lost your memory?	☐	☐
33. Have you ever had a seizure?	☐	☐
34. Do you have headaches with exercise?	☐	☐
35. Have you ever had numbness, tingling, or weakness in your arms or legs after being hit or falling?	☐	☐
36. Have you ever been unable to move your arms or legs after being hit or falling?	☐	☐
37. When exercising in the heat, do you have severe muscle cramps or become ill?	☐	☐
38. Has a doctor told you that you or someone in your family has sickle cell trait or sickle cell disease?	☐	☐
39. Have you had any problems with your eyes or vision?	☐	☐
40. Do you wear glasses or contact lenses?	☐	☐
41. Do you wear protective eyewear, such as goggles or a face shield?	☐	☐
42. Are you happy with your weight?	☐	☐
43. Are you trying to gain or lose weight?	☐	☐
44. Has anyone recommended you change your weight or eating habits?	☐	☐
45. Do you limit or carefully control what you eat?	☐	☐
46. Do you have any concerns that you would like to discuss with a doctor?	☐	☐

FEMALES ONLY

	Yes	No
47. Have you ever had a menstrual period?	☐	☐

48. How old were you when you had your first menstrual period?_____
49. How many periods have you had in the last year?_____

Explain "Yes" answers here:_____
_____
_____
_____
_____
_____
_____
_____

I hereby state that, to the best of my knowledge, my answers to the above questions are complete and correct.

Signature of athlete _____ Signature of parent/guardian _____ Date _____

© 2004 *American Academy of Family Physicians, American Academy of Pediatrics, American College of Sports Medicine, American Medical Society for Sports Medicine, American Orthopaedic Society for Sports Medicine, and American Osteopathic Academy of Sports Medicine.*

Fig. 1. Sample history form. (*From* The Physician and Sportsmedicine. Preparticipation physical evaluation, 3rd edition. Elk Grove Village, IL:American Academy of Pediatrics, 2004; with permission.)

All allergies, including drug, contact, and food allergy, should be documented. Serious allergic reactions to food or insect stings may occur during team travel. Availability and dosing indications of diphenhydramine and injectable epinephrine should be discussed with the team staff as needed.

Preparticipation Physical Evaluation   PHYSICAL EXAMINATION FORM

Name _____ Date of birth _____

Height _____ Weight _____ % Body fat (optional) _____ Pulse_____ BP___/____ (___/___ , ___/___)

Vision R 20/ _____ L 20/ _____   Corrected: Y N   Pupils: Equal _____ Unequal _____

Follow-Up Questions on More Sensitive Issues	Yes	No
1. Do you feel stressed out or under a lot of pressure?	☐	☐
2. Do you ever feel so sad or hopeless that you stop doing some of your usual activities for more than a few days?	☐	☐
3. Do you feel safe?	☐	☐
4. Have you ever tried cigarette smoking, even 1 or 2 puffs? Do you currently smoke?	☐	☐
5. During the past 30 days, did you use chewing tobacco, snuff, or dip?	☐	☐
6. During the past 30 days, have you had at least 1 drink of alcohol?	☐	☐
7. Have you ever taken steroid pills or shots without a doctor's prescription?	☐	☐
8. Have you ever taken any supplements to help you gain or lose weight or improve your performance?	☐	☐
9. Questions from the Youth Risk Behavior Survey (http://www.cdc.gov/HealthyYouth/yrbs/index.htm) on guns, seatbelts, unprotected sex, domestic violence, drugs, etc	☐	☐

Notes: _____
_____
_____

	NORMAL	ABNORMAL FINDINGS	INITIALS*
MEDICAL			
Appearance			
Eyes/ears/nose/throat			
Hearing			
Lymph nodes			
Heart			
Murmurs			
Pulses			
Lungs			
Abdomen			
Genitourinary†			
Skin			
MUSCULOSKELETAL			
Neck			
Back			
Shoulder/arm			
Elbow/forearm			
Wrist/hand/fingers			
Hip/thigh			
Knee			
Leg/ankle			
Foot/toes			

*Multiple-examiner set-up only.
†Having a third party present is recommended for the genitourinary examination.

Notes: _____
_____

Name of physician (print/type)_____ Date _____

Address _____ Phone _____

Signature of physician_____, MD or DO

Fig. 1 (*continued*)

Cardiovascular history

In the United States, the incidence of sudden cardiac death in high school athletes is between 1:100,000 and 1:300,000 [7,8]. The goal of the PPE is to identify high-risk athletes thorough a comprehensive family history, review

Preparticipation Physical Evaluation

CLEARANCE FORM

Name_____ Sex_____ Age_____ Date of birth_____

❏ Cleared without restriction

❏ Cleared, with recommendations for further evaluation or treatment for: _____

_____

_____

_____

❏ Not cleared for ❏ All sports ❏ Certain sports: _____ Reason: _____

Recommendations: _____

_____

EMERGENCY INFORMATION

Allergies_____

Other Information _____

IMMUNIZATIONS (eg, tetanus/diphtheria; measles, mumps, rubella; hepatitis A, B; influenza; poliomyelitis; pneumococcal; meningococcal; varicella)

❏ Up to date (see attached documentation) ❏ Not up to date Specify _____

Name of physician (print/type) _____ Date _____

Address _____ Phone_____

Signature of physician _____, MD or DO

© 2004 *American Academy of Family Physicians, American Academy of Pediatrics, American Medical Society for Sports Medicine, American Orthopaedic Society for Sports Medicine, and American Osteopathic Academy of Sports Medicine.*

Preparticipation Physical Evaluation

CLEARANCE FORM

Name_____ Sex_____ Age_____ Date of birth_____

❏ Cleared without restriction

❏ Cleared, with recommendations for further evaluation or treatment for: _____

_____

_____

_____

❏ Not cleared for ❏ All sports ❏ Certain sports: _____ Reason: _____

Recommendations: _____

_____

EMERGENCY INFORMATION

Allergies_____

Other Information _____

IMMUNIZATIONS (eg, tetanus/diphtheria; measles, mumps, rubella; hepatitis A, B; influenza; poliomyelitis; pneumococcal; meningococcal; varicella)

❏ Up to date (see attached documentation) ❏ Not up to date Specify _____

Name of physician (print/type) _____ Date _____

Address _____ Phone_____

Signature of physician _____, MD or DO

© 2004 *American Academy of Family Physicians, American Academy of Pediatrics, American Medical Society for Sports Medicine, American Orthopaedic Society for Sports Medicine, and American Osteopathic Academy of Sports Medicine.*

Fig. 1 (*continued*)

of symptoms, and physical examination. The American Heart Association has developed a series of recommendations (Box 1) to help identify at-risk athletes [9]. The examiner focuses on the athlete's history of heart murmur, syncope or presyncope, exertional chest pain, easy fatigability, and palpitations. Symptomatic individuals require further evaluation. Athletes who have a family history of sudden cardiac death in relatives under the age of 50, hypertrophic cardiomyopathy, Marfan's syndrome, or inheritable arrhythmias also warrant a full cardiac evaluation. Routine echocardiograms and electrocardiograms in asymptomatic athletes are not recommended at the high school level [9].

Respiratory

The incidence of asthma in the general pediatric population is 6.7% (1:15) [10], and up to 19% of nonasthmatic individuals may experience exercise-induced bronchospasm (EIB) under certain conditions [11]. Appropriate questions include shortness of breath with exercise, wheezing, poor exercise tolerance, or coughing associated with exercise. Unfortunately, history and symptoms alone are poor (45%) predictors of a correct diagnosis [10]. Field testing under real conditions with hand-held incentive spirometer provides more objective data. History should focus on prior severe EIB episodes, hospitalizations or emergency room visits, recent asthma control, and current treatment.

Concussion/head/neck injury

In high school football, the documented rate of mild traumatic brain injury (concussion) is about 5% per year [12]. Recent evidence suggests that adolescent brains recover slower that adult brains [13]. History should document the total number of concussions, the recovery time from each concussion, and presence of postconcussive symptoms. History also should include past imaging (MRI) and completion of neuropsychological testing.

Brachial plexus injuries, called burners or stingers, are common in collision sports. A positive history requires careful upper extremity examination and possibly further imaging. A history of bilateral upper and/or lower extremity neurologic symptoms requires further evaluation for serious conditions such as spinal cord stenosis or cervical instability.

Orthopedic history

The history should focus on injuries that resulted in missed practices or games, or required surgery. The physician should inquire about rehabilitation history, current functional deficits, and any braces or special devices used now or in the past. Information obtained during the history will guide and focus the physical examination.

Heat illness

Every year, many high school athletes suffer from a spectrum of heat-related illnesses. There are several factors than must be considered when evaluating athletes who participate in hot and humid environments. Sickle cell trait [14], obesity, and poor conditioning are known risk factors for heat illness. Over-the-counter stimulants, methylphenidate, antihistamines and anticholinergics, second-generation neuroleptics, selected selective serotonin reuptake inhibitors (SSRIs) and diuretics also may increase risk to heat illness. The physical maturity level of the athlete also is

Table 2
Medical conditions and sports participation*

Condition	May participate
Atlantoaxial instability (instability of the joint between cervical vertebrae 1 and 2)	Qualified yes
Explanation: Athlete needs evaluation to assess risk of spinal cord injury during sports participation.	
Bleeding disorder	Qualified yes
Explanation: Athlete needs evaluation.	
Cardiovascular disease	
Carditis (inflammation of the heart)	No
Explanation: Carditis may result in sudden death with exertion.	
Hypertension (high blood pressure)	Qualified yes
Explanation: Those with significant essential (unexplained) hypertension should avoid weight and power lifting, body building, and strength training. Those with secondary hypertension (hypertension caused by a previously identified disease) or severe essential hypertension need evaluation. The National High Blood Pressure Education Working group defined significant and severe hypertension.	
Congenital heart disease (structural heart defects present at birth)	Qualified yes
Explanation: Those with mild forms may participate fully; those with moderate or severe forms or who have undergone surgery need evaluation. The 26th Bethesda Conference defined mild, moderate, and severe disease for common cardiac lesions.	
Dysrhythmia (irregular heart rhythm)	Qualified yes
Explanation: Those with symptoms (chest pain, syncope, dizziness, shortness of breath, or other symptoms of possible dysrhythmia) or evidence of mitral regurgitation (leaking) on physical examination need evaluation. All others may participate fully	
Heart murmur	Qualified yes
Explanation: If the murmur is innocent (does not indicate heart disease), full participation is permitted. Otherwise, the athlete needs evaluation (see congenital heart disease and mitral valve prolapse).	
Cerebral palsy	Qualified yes
Explanation: Athlete needs evaluation.	
Diabetes mellitus	Yes
Explanation: All sports can be played with proper attention to diet, blood glucose concentration, hydration, and insulin therapy. Blood glucose concentration should be monitored every 30 minutes during continuous exercise and 15 minutes after completion of exercise.	
Diarrhea	Qualified no
Explanation: Unless disease is mild, no participation is permitted, because diarrhea may increase the risk of dehydration and heat illness. See fever.	

(continued on next page)

Table 2 (*continued*)

Condition	May participate
Eating disorders	Qualified yes
Anorexia nervosa	
Bulimia nervosa	
Explanation: Patients with these disorders need medical and psychiatric assessment before participation.	
Eyes	Qualified yes
Functionally one-eyed athlete	
Loss of an eye	
Detached retina	
Previous eye surgery or serious eye injury	
Explanation: A functionally one-eyed athlete has a best-corrected visual acuity of less than 20/40 in the eye with worse acuity. These athletes would suffer significant disability if the better eye were seriously injured, as would those with loss of an eye. Some athletes who previously have undergone eye surgery or had a serious eye injury may have an increased risk of injury because of weakened eye tissue. Availability of eye guards approved by the American Society for Testing and Materials and other protective equipment may allow participation in most sports, but this must be judged on an individual basis.	
Fever	No
Explanation: Fever can increase cardiopulmonary effort, reduce maximum exercise capacity, make heat illness more likely, and increase orthostatic hypertension during exercise. Fever may rarely accompany myocarditis or other infections that may make exercise dangerous.	
Heat illness, history of	Qualified yes
Explanation: Because of the increased likelihood of recurrence, the athlete needs individual assessment to determine the presence of predisposing conditions and to arrange a prevention strategy.	
Hepatitis	Yes
Explanation: Because of the apparent minimal risk to others, all sports may be played that the athlete's state of health allows. In all athletes, skin lesions should be covered properly, and athletic personnel should use universal precautions when handling blood or body fluids with visible blood.	
Human immunodeficiency virus infection	Yes
Explanation: Because of the apparent minimal risk to others, all sports may be played that the athlete's state of health allows. In all athletes, skin lesions should be covered properly, and athletic personnel should use universal precautions when handling blood or body fluids with visible blood.	
Kidney, absence of one	Qualified yes
Explanation: Athlete needs individual assessment for contact, collision, and limited-contact sports.	

(*continued on next page*)

Table 2 *(continued)*

Condition	May participate
Liver, enlarged	Qualified yes
Explanation: If the liver is acutely enlarged, participation should be avoided because of risk of rupture. If the liver is chronically enlarged, individual assessment is needed before collision, contact, or limited-contact sports are played.	
Malignant neoplasm	Qualified yes
Explanation: Athlete needs individual assessment.	
Musculoskeletal disorders	Qualified yes
Explanation: Athlete needs individual assessment.	
Neurologic disorders	
History of serious head or spine trauma, severe or repeated concussions, or crainotomy.	Qualified yes
Explanation: Athlete needs individual assessment for collision, contact, or limited-contact sports and also for noncontact sports if deficits in judgment or cognition are present. Research supports a conservative approach to management of concussion.	
Seizure disorder, well-controlled	Yes
Explanation: Risk of seizure during participation is minimal	
Seizure disorder, poorly controlled	Qualified yes
Explanation: Athlete needs individual assessment for collision, contact, or limited-contact sports. The following noncontact sports should be avoided: archery, riflery, swimming, weight or power lifting, strength training, or sports involving heights. In these sports, occurrence of a seizure may pose a risk to self or others.	
Obesity	Qualified yes
Explanation: Because of the risk of heat illness, obese persons need careful acclimatization and hydration.	
Organ transplant recipient	Qualified yes
Explanation: Athlete needs individual assessment.	
Ovary, absence of one	Yes
Explanation: Risk of severe injury to the remaining ovary is minimal.	
Respiratory conditions	
Pulmonary compromise, including cystic fibrosis	Qualified yes
Explanation: Athlete needs individual assessment, but generally, all sports may be played if oxygenation remains satisfactory during a graded exercise test. Patients with cystic fibrosis need acclimatization and good hydration to reduce the risk of heat illness.	
Asthma	Yes
Explanation: With proper medication and education, only athletes with the most severe asthma will need to modify their participation.	
Acute upper respiratory infection	Qualified yes
Explanation: Upper respiratory obstruction may affect pulmonary function. Athlete needs individual assessment for all but mild disease. See fever.	

(continued on next page)

Table 2 (*continued*)

Condition	May participate
Sickle cell disease	Qualified yes
Explanation: Athlete needs individual assessment. In general, if status of the illness permits, all but high exertion, collision, and contact sports may be played. Overheating, dehydration, and chilling must be avoided.	
Sickle cell trait	Yes
Explanation: It is unlikely that persons with sickle cell trait have an increased risk of sudden death or other medical problems during athletic participation, except under the most extreme conditions of heat, humidity, and possibly increased altitude. These persons, like all athletes, should be carefully conditioned, acclimatized, and hydrated to reduce any possible risk.	
Skin disorders (boils, herpes simplex, impetigo, scabies, molluscum contagiosum)	Qualified yes
Explanation: While the patient is contagious, participation in gymnastics with mats; martial arts; wrestling; or other collision, contact, or limited-contact sports is not allowed.	
Spleen, enlarged	Qualified yes
Explanation: A patient with an acutely enlarged spleen should avoid all sports because of risk of rupture. A patient with a chronically enlarged spleen needs individual assessment before playing collision, contact, or limited-contact sports.	
Testicle, undescended or absence of one	Yes
Explanation: Certain sports may require a protective cup.	

* This table is designed for use by medical and nonmedical personnel. "Needs evaluation" means that a physician with appropriate knowledge and experience should assess the safety of a given sport for an athlete with the listed medical condition. Unless otherwise noted, this is because of variability of the severity of the disease, the risk of injury for the specific sports.

Adapted from Committee on Sports Medicine and Fitness. American Academy of Pediatrics: Medical conditions affecting sports participation. Pediatrics 2001;107(5):1205–9; with permission.

a consideration. Children are more at risk for exertional heat illness than adults, as their thermoregulation centers are less developed. Children initiate sweating at higher core temperatures and have a delayed thirst response to mild dehydration. Children have fewer sweat glands and produce small volumes of sweat per gland. Their increased body surface area results in increased environmental heat gain on hot days. Young athletes also take longer to acclimate to heat than adults [15]. Individuals who have identifiable risks should be counseled on heat illness signs and symptoms while coaches and medical staffs increase their vigilance.

Menstrual history and nutrition

Athletes at risk for disordered eating should be screened with general questions of ideal weight and satisfaction with current weight. An abnormal menstrual history in female athletes (oligo-or amenorrhea) may suggest

---

Box 1. American Heart Association recommendations to identify risk of sudden cardiac death in athletes

Screening review of systems:
Does the athlete experience chest pain, shortness of breath, or abnormal heart beats during exercise?
Has the athlete ever experienced syncope or near syncope during or after exercise?
Is there a recent history of unexplained exercise intolerance (a change in the ability to normally keep up with peers)

Screening history:
Does the athlete have any history of heart murmur or hypertension or any cardiac conditions?
Has the athlete ever had any cardiac testing including ECG or echocardiogram?
Is there a family history of sudden or unexplained death in relative less than age 50?
Is there anyone in the family under age 50 with heart disease?
Is there anyone in the family with known heart conditions, including hypertrophic cardiomyopathy, Marfan's syndrome, long QT, or other arrhythmogenic disorders?

Screening physical examination:
Take sitting blood pressure.
Auscultate heart in two positions (supine and seated/standing).
Check femoral pulses.
Evaluate for physical signs of Marfan's syndrome.

Adapted from Recommendations and considerations related to preparticipation screening for cardiovascular abnormalities in competitive athletes: 2007 update. Circulation 2007;115:1643–55; with permission.

---

inadequate caloric intake. Menstrual irregularities are common in adolescent females. Menstrual cycle lengths outside the 95th percentile (90 days for the first year, 50 days by the fourth year) should be evaluated [16].

Physical examination

The physical examination should focus on the organ systems most pertinent for safe participation, namely, the cardiovascular, neurologic, and musculoskeletal systems.

Vital signs

Height, weight, pulse, a seated blood pressure and corrected vision screening are standard for the PPE. Height and weight should be compared with age- and sex-adjusted norms as necessary. Body fat percentage may be required for wrestlers. Dramatic weight loss should arouse suspicion for disordered eating.

Head, eyes, ears, nose, throat

The examination specifically should document absent teeth, differences in pupil size (physiologic anisocoria), cranial nerve abnormalities, and any other relevant issues. Smokeless tobacco use necessitates careful evaluation of the oral mucosa.

Cardiovascular

Physical examination includes assessment of pulses, auscultation, and assessment for characteristics of Marfan's syndrome (Box 2). Murmurs that necessitate further evaluation include moderate intensity (3/6) and louder, diastolic murmurs, and any murmur that increases in intensity with decreases in cardiac preload (sitting-to-standing, Valsalva maneuver).

Abdomen/Genitourinary

Examination should document any hepatomegaly, splenomegaly, or testicular abnormalities (males only). In females, pregnancy may be suspected if the uterus is palpable in the lower abdomen.

Skin

The skin examination is essential for wrestling or other sports where active infection prohibits participation. Infections such as herpes gladiatorum, molluscum contagiosum, and bacterial infections (impetigo) are common in these sports and require deferred clearance when present.

Box 2. Physical characteristics of Marfan's syndrome

Arachnodactyly
Arm span > height
Thumb sign
Wrist sign
Kyphosis
High arched palate
Pectus excavatum
Mitral valve prolapse
Myopia
Lenticular dislocation
Aortic insufficiency

Musculoskeletal

The standard PPE should include a basic screening orthopedic examination (Box 3). Individuals should be clothed appropriately to allow a full inspection of the upper and lower extremities, including the shoulders, and the back/chest as indicated. Any joint with a history of previous injury will require a more detailed examination that includes range of motion, ligament stability testing, muscle strength testing, presence or absence of joint effusion, documentation of any soft tissue or bony tenderness, and a thorough neurovascular examination.

Special testing

As this time, the consensus statement from the major sports medicine associations in the United States does not recommended any laboratory testing to be part of the standard preparticipation evaluation [17]. In Europe, screening electrocardiograms are often part of a sports evaluation, but the American Heart Association does not recommend screening electrocardiograms or screening echocardiograms for high school athletes in the United States [9,18].

Clearance

Final clearance decisions should be based on the following questions. First, does participation put the athlete at risk for serious injury or illness? Does participation place other participants at risk for injury or illness? Finally, can the risks of participation be modified by available treatments

---

Box 3. Screening orthopedic examination

Upper extremity testing
Neck ROM: turn head left, right, up, down, ear to ipsilateral
  shoulder
Shoulder ROM: forward flexion, abduction, with arms at 90
  degrees abduction check internal/external rotation
Elbow: flexion, extension
Wrist: pronation, supination, flexion, extension
Hand: spread fingers, make a fist
Spine: Forward bend at waist- look for rib hump consistent with
  scoliosis, extension at waist

Lower extremity testing
Squat like a baseball catcher, Duck walk, toe walk, normal gait,
  single leg hop

(athletic equipment/medicines)? Can modified participation be allowed while treatment is started?

Clearance must take into account the limitations of the athlete's condition and the demands of the sport. An athlete may be cleared for some activities (clearance with restrictions) and not cleared for others. Clearance also may change over time as injuries are rehabilitated or medical conditions improve. Final clearance decisions must weigh various factors to make decisions that are in the best interest of the athlete.

Common clearance issues

Orthopedic

Orthopedic history and physical examination findings present the most common clearance issues to the examiner. Factors to be considered include the current status of an injury and the demands of the particular sport. Criteria for clearance include full range of motion of the involved joint, symmetric strength, and normal joint stability. Deferred clearance may be indicated to more fully rehabilitate a given condition before the start of training and competition.

Cardiovascular

Hypertension in the adolescent athlete is defined as three consecutive readings greater than 95% on age-, height-, and sex-adjusted graphs. Evaluation of all hypertensive adolescents should include a urine analysis, urine culture, complete blood cell count, basic metabolic panel, fasting glucose and lipid panels, renal ultrasound, echocardiogram, and retinal examination to evaluate for end organ damage. Athletes who have stage 1 hypertension (Table 3) may continue to participate in sports while evaluation is ongoing. Athletes who have stage 2 hypertension require full evaluation and control of blood pressure before clearance [19].

Clearance for athletes who have significant structural or electrical abnormalities can present significant challenges to the sports medicine physician. In general, decision-making for myocardial disorders, valvular problems, and arrhythmias should follow the 36th Bethesda Conference guidelines [18]. Unique circumstances, however, may dictate deviation from these guidelines on rare occasion.

Table 3
Classification of hypertension

Stage 1 hypertension	Stage 2 hypertension
Pediatrics: blood pressure (BP) between 95% and 99% plus 5 mm Hg and no evidence of end organ damage	Pediatrics: BP greater than 99% plus 5 mm Hg or hypertension with end organ damage
Adults: BP between 140/90 and 159/99	Adults: BP greater than 160/100

Neurologic

Recovery from a mild traumatic brain injury in the high school athlete is delayed compared with recovery in college and adult athletes [13,20]. Athletes who have sustained multiple concussions or experienced prolonged postconcussive symptoms require careful evaluation before clearance for contact and collision sports. Clearance is deferred for athletes who are experiencing ongoing postconcussive symptoms. Athletes should be symptom-free at rest and during exercise before being cleared to return to sports [21]. Neuropsychological testing is used commonly at all levels of competition and may be aid in the evaluation process.

A history of transient quadriparesis requires consultation before clearance for contact and collision sports. Clearance for athletes diagnosed with cervical stenosis is somewhat controversial and deserves careful and individualized attention. Athletes who have well-controlled seizure disorders may compete in most sports including collision sports. Participation in sports where a seizure could be life-threatening to either the athlete or to other competitors, such as rock climbing, archery, or riflery, is not recommended [22,23].

Single paired organs

Athletes who have a single parted organ (eye, testicle) may compete with protective equipment after a full and complete discussion of the risks of participation. Some controversy exists regarding athletes who have a single kidney participating in contact and collision sports. The scientific literature suggests that the risks of serious injury to a kidney are far less then the risks of a sudden cardiac event [24]. Participation should be discussed in a multi-disciplinary group with the athlete, parents, and physician(s) knowledgeable of the risks before clearance.

Legal issues

State or local laws frequently mandate the preparticipation evaluation before athletic competition. Federal regulations, however, govern the laws regarding health information and patient confidentiality. The Health Insurance Portability and Accountability Act (HIPPA) applies to examinations done in a private setting. In mass school screenings, the Family Education Rights and Privacy Act (FERPA) guidelines usually are applicable. Although the FERPA guidelines allow public school employees, including school nurses, school physicians, athletic trainers, and coaches, to share medically necessary information, the HIPPA guidelines do not. During competition, the athletic trainer or coach will be the first responder to any medical problems. Athletic trainers frequently hold medical supplies such as albuterol inhalers, epinephrine pens, or insulin for the athletes during competition. Therefore, it is in the best interest of the athlete that coaches and athletic trainers are aware of medically relevant issues. In the context of the PPE, the private physician should obtain consent from the adolescent and guardian to discuss relevant medical information with the team staff.

References

[1] National Federation of State High School Associations (NFHS). 2005–2006 high school athletics participation survey. Indianapolis (IN): NHFS; 2006. Available at: http://www.nfhs.org/sports.aspx.

[2] Krowchuk DP, Krowchuk HV, Hunter DM, et al. Parents' knowledge of the purposes and content of preparticipation physical examinations. Arch Pediatr Adolesc Med 1995;149(6): 653–7.

[3] DuRant RH, Seymore C, Linder CW, et al. The preparticipation examination of athletes: comparison of single and multiple examiners. Am J Dis Child 1985;139:657–61.

[4] Riser WL, Hoffman HM, Bellah GG Jr. Frequency of preparticipation sports examinations in secondary school athletes: are the University Interscholastic League guidelines appropriate? Tex Med 1985;81(7):35–9.

[5] Goldberg B, Saraniti A, Whitman P, et al. Preparticipation sports assessment: an objective evaluation. Pediatrics 1980;66(5):736–45.

[6] Kowatari K, Nakashima K, Ono A, et al. Leovofloxacin-induced bilateral Achilles tendon rupture: a case report and review of the literature. J Orthop Sci 2004;9(2):186–90.

[7] Maron BJ, Shirani J, Poliac LC, et al. Sudden death in young competitive athletes: clinical, demographic, and pathological profiles. JAMA 1996;276(3):199–204.

[8] Van Camp SP, Bloor CM, Mueller FO, et al. Nontraumatic sports deaths in high school and college athletes. Med Sci Sports Exerc 1995;27(5):641–7.

[9] Marion BJ, Maron B, Thompson PJ, et al. Considerations related to preparticipation screening for cardiovascular abnormalities in competitive athletes: 2007 update. Circulation 2007; 115:1643–55.

[10] National Asthma Education and Prevention Program. Expert panel report: guidelines for the diagnosis and management of asthma: update on selected topics 2002. Bethesda (MD): National Institutes of Health; 2003, Publication #NIH 02-5074.

[11] Rundell KW, Jenkinson DM. Exercise-induced bronchospasm in the elite athlete. Sports Med 2002;32:583–600.

[12] Guskiewicz KM, Weaver NL, Padua DA, et al. Epidemiology of concussion in collegiate and high school football players. Am J Sports Med 2000;28:643–50.

[13] Field M, Collins MW, Lovell MR, et al. Does age play a role in recovery from sports-related concussion? A comparison of high school and collegiate athletes. J Pediatr 2003;142(5): 546–53.

[14] Kark JA, Posey DM, Schumacher HR, et al. Sickle cell trait as a risk factor for sudden death in physical training. N Engl J Med 1987;317(13):781–7.

[15] American Academy of Pediatrics Committee on Sports Medicine and Fitness: climatic heat stress and the exercising child and adolescent. Pediatrics 2000;106:158–9.

[16] AAP clinical report: menstruation in girls and adolescents: using the menstrual cycle as a vital sign. Pediatrics 2006;118(5):2245–50.

[17] American Academy of Family Physicians, American Academy of Pediatrics, American College of Sports Medicine, American Medical Society for Sports Medicine, American Orthopaedic Society for Sports Medicine, American Osteopathic Academy of Sports Medicine. Preparticipation physical evaluation. 3rd edition. McGraw-Hill; 2005. p. 8–9.

[18] 36th Bethesda Conference. Eligibility recommendations for competitive athletes with cardio-vascular abnormalities: November 6, 2004. J Am Coll Cardiol 2005;45:1317–75.

[19] National High Blood Pressure Education Program Working Group on High Blood Pressure in Children and Adolescents. The fourth report on the diagnosis, evaluation, and treatment of high blood pressure in children and adolescents. Pediatrics 2004;114:555–76.

[20] Kirkwood MW, Yeates KO, Wilson PE. Pediatric sport-related concussion: a review of the clinical management of an oft-neglected population. Pediatrics 2006;117(4):1359–71.

[21] McCrory P, Johnston K, Meeuwisse W, et al. Summary and agreement statement of the Second International Conference on Concussion in Sports, Prague 2004. Physician and Sports Medicine 2005;33:29–40.

[22] Fountain NB, May AC. Epilepsy and athletics. Clin Sports Med 2003;22(3):605–16.

[23] Dubow JS, Kelly JP. Epilepsy in sports and recreation. Sports Med 2003;33(7):499–516.

[24] Grinsell MM, Showalter S, Gordon KA, et al. Single kidney and sports participation: perception versus reality. Pediatrics 2006;118(3):1019–27.

ELSEVIER
SAUNDERS

Phys Med Rehabil Clin N Am
19 (2008) 235–245

PHYSICAL MEDICINE
AND REHABILITATION
CLINICS OF
NORTH AMERICA

Strength Training Recommendations for the Young Athlete

Jeffrey M. Vaughn, DO[a],*, Lyle Micheli, MD[a,b]

[a]Division of Sports Medicine, Boston Children's Hospital, 319 Longwood Avenue,
Boston, MA 02115, USA
[b]Harvard Medical School, 319 Longwood Avenue, Boston, MA 02115, USA

Over the past two decades, recommendations for strength training in youth have made pivotal changes in response to several studies that have given us new understanding regarding the safety and efficacy of strength training in the prepubescent athlete [1–6]. Not only have many of the concerns over subjecting the immature skeleton to repetitive loading been resolved [6–8], many of the benefits gained from youth resistance training have been substantiated [9–12]. Strength training has become recognized as an effective method to help youth enjoy sports by decreasing their risk of injury [9,10,13,14] and increasing their chance of success by improving their performance [10,15,16].

Some of the issues that have been addressed in recent studies of resistance training in preadolescent athletes include: the appropriate age for strength training, neuromuscular adaptations, training frequency, number of repetitions, and detraining. The purpose of this article is to present the most current recommendations for strength training in the preadolescent athlete and to provide guidelines that can be used in developing a program that is both safe and effective.

Age

The first consideration involving age is whether strength training is safe for the prepubescent athlete. Much of this concern is related to the open physis. Because cartilage is weaker than bone, many have considered the physis to be the "weak link" in the skeleton. Their concern has been that placing the physis under superphysiologic and repetitive loads would

---

* Corresponding author.
E-mail address: jeffrey.vaughn@childrens.harvard.edu (J.M. Vaughn).

1047-9651/08/$ - see front matter © 2008 Elsevier Inc. All rights reserved.
doi:10.1016/j.pmr.2007.11.004

pmr.theclinics.com

potentially damage the physis, causing it to prematurely fuse, resulting in limb deformity and cessation of limb growth [9,10]. Micheli [1] noted, however, that the potential for a growth plate injury may actually be less in a child than in an adolescent because the epiphyseal plate of a child is stronger and more resistant to shearing forces.

The few studies that have reported injuries to the epiphyseal plate from strength training have been in adolescents and have been attributed to improper lifting techniques, lifting maximal amounts of weights, and lifts performed without adequate adult supervision [17]. Growth plate injuries have not been reported in any prospective resistance training study that included prescribed training regimens and competent instruction [10]. To protect the growth plate from potential injury, it is recommended that children avoid improper lifting techniques and never perform heavy lifts in an unsupervised setting [9].

The second issue related to the age a child should begin strength training concerns the efficacy of strength training in children. Because prepubertal boys do not have sufficient levels of circulating androgens to allow for muscles to hypertrophy in response to weight training, in the past it was believed that they could not benefit from weight training.

In 1978, a study by Vrijens questioned whether preadolescents could gain any benefit from weight training [18]. In a group of six boys with an average age of 10.4 years, no significant increase in strength or muscle cross-sectional area was noted after 8 weeks of strength training. When assessed in the light of recent strength studies in children, it seems these findings were likely the result of a low training volume and intensity. In this same vein, a position paper by the American Academy of Pediatrics in 1983 stated that "prepubertal boys do not significantly improve strength or improve muscle mass in a weight training program because of insufficient levels of circulating androgens" [19].

One of the earliest articles demonstrating the effectiveness of strength training in preadolescents was a study by Sewall and Micheli [2]. In this study 18 prepubescent children strength trained three times per week for 9 weeks. Mean strength increase was 42.9%, compared with an increase of only 9.5% in the control group. Ramsay attributed these gains in strength to adaptations in muscle excitation-contraction coupling, increased motor unit activation, and improved motor skill coordination [3].

Within the last 10 years, clinical studies and observations have confirmed that a resistance training program of sufficient duration and intensity can enhance the strength of prepubescents beyond what it is as a result of normal growth and development [10]. Although the earliest age that a child should be involved in strength training has yet to be determined, all participants should have the emotional maturity to accept and follow directions, and should understand both the benefits and risks associated with strength training [9]. In a report by Falk [20], children as young as 6 years old benefited from weight training.

Training frequency

The American College of Sports Medicine recommends that children strength train two to three times per week on nonconsecutive days [10]. Too much exercise may lead to overuse injuries by not allowing adequate time for musculoskeletal tissues to recover between training episodes [7]. Too little strength training may lead to loss of the strength gained during a period of training [2,21]. To avoid overuse injury, Micheli recommended allowing adequate recovery time between training sessions and not advancing the volume or intensity of training too soon [7,17].

Several studies have supported the recommendation of strength training several days per week. Faigenbaum [22] showed that larger strength gains can be made by children performing strength training twice per week as compared with once per week. After 8 weeks of strength training, children (aged 7–12) that trained twice per week had increased their one repetition maximum (1RM) on the chest press by 11.5%, compared with 9% by those who worked out only once per week and 4.4% in the control group. In the leg press, a 24.9% increase in the 1RM was observed by those who worked out twice per week, compared with a 14.2% and 2.4% increase in those who worked out once per week and the control group, respectively. In an additional study by Faigenbaum and colleagues [23], boys and girls between the ages of 8 and 12 increased their strength an average of 74.3%, compared with 13.0% in the control group after 8 weeks of performing three sets of five different exercises twice per week.

Repetitions

A few studies have examined the influence of exercise volume on strength gains in children. In 1999 Faigenbaum and colleagues [4] performed a study comparing a group of 15 children, strength training using a heavy load and performing one set of six to eight repetitions (low repetition-heavy load), to a group of children training with a moderate load and performing one set of 13 to 15 repetitions (high repetition-moderate load). Participants were assigned to strength train twice per week for a total of 8 weeks. The high repetition-moderate load group was found to have a significantly higher increase in strength (40.9% compared with 31.0%) than the low repetition-heavy load group.

An additional study performed in 2001 by Faigenbaum and colleagues [24] lent support to his previous findings that using a higher number of repetitions with a moderate load led to greater strength gains than training with a heavier load and performing a lower number of repetitions. This study divided children into groups performing four different resistance-training protocols. The first group performed six to eight repetitions on the chest press with a heavy load. A second group performed 13 to 15 repetitions of the same exercise with a moderate load. A third group performed six to eight repetitions of chest press, immediately followed by six to eight medicine ball chest passes (12–16 total repetitions), and a fourth group performing only one set of 13 to 15 medicine ball chest passes. The only groups who improved their strength (using a 1RM chest press strength) after an 8-week training program were the groups who performed a higher number of repetitions and used the chest press as part of their training protocol.

The number of repetitions a child is able to perform often varies between exercises and is most likely the result of differing amounts of muscle mass involved in each exercise [25]. In a study using percentages of the 1RM it was found that the number of repetitions a child could perform at a specific percentage of the 1RM varied between exercises [26]. The number of repetitions that each child could perform at a given percentage of the 1RM was significantly greater when performing the leg press than when performing the chest press.

The method used by Dr. Thomas DeLorme to determine effectual ratios of resistance to repetitions for young military males in a rehabilitation setting is still used today in many training centers [27]. The 1RM was determined each week. The patient then trained at 60% to 70% of the 1RM, while usually closely approximating the 10RM, depending on the lift being performed. Concerns have been raised, however, regarding the safety of performing the one repetition maximum in children.

Perhaps the safest way to determine the number or repetitions that should be performed for each exercise in children is by starting with a relatively low weight that a child can easily lift 13 to 15 times without difficulty, and then increasing the weight until a point where a child is able to perform no more than 15 repetitions, but is able to perform at least 13 repetitions. As the child's strength increases, the amount of weight he or she is lifting can be increased by 2.5 to 5 pounds until the number of repetitions they can perform is within a set number of repetitions [9,11].

Single versus multiple sets

Whether a single set is as efficient in making strength gains as performing multiple sets of the same exercise has been the subject of several studies and meta-analysis [28–30] in the adult population; however, no studies have been performed specific to the preadolescent athlete. Recent studies in adult populations support greater strength gains when using multiple sets rather than single sets, especially after progression occurs and higher gains are desired [29].

In a study by Rhea and colleagues [28], young men (age 21, plus or minus 2 years) were randomized to groups performing one or three sets of leg presses and bench presses, three times a week for a period of 12 weeks. Using 1RM testing, those in the group performing three sets of each exercise made 30% greater strength gains in the leg press and 13% greater strength gains in the bench press than those performing only one set of each exercise.

Similar findings were seen in a study [30] performed in a group of women performing either one or three sets of a variety of exercises for a period of 6 weeks.

Currently, the National Strength and Conditioning Association supports preadolescents performing one to three sets of a variety of single- and multi-joint exercises [10]. Increasing the number of sets performed is another way to influence an athlete's strength progression. Further studies conducted in preadolescents may provide additional information regarding whether the number of sets performed on each exercise effects strength gains.

Rest period between sets

The time an athlete should rest between sets to get the most out of his or her training has been the subject of various studies in adult populations [31–34]. No study in preadolescents has specifically addressed this subject.

In a study by Richmond and Godard [31], 28 men performed two sets of bench presses to volitional exhaustion. Rest periods of 1, 3, and 5 minutes between sets were used on three separate testing days. No difference in total work load (repetitions × weight) was found between the 3- and 5- minute rest periods, but the work load decreased significantly if the rest period was decreased to 1 minute.

Hill-Haas and colleagues [32], found a greater increase in strength (45.9% versus 19.6%) after a 5 week strength training program in women given an 80-second rest interval between sets, compared with those given a 20-second rest interval.

Although trying to manipulate as many variables as possible to get as much as possible out of a strength training session may be a prudent use of time, structuring a workout program too rigidly may discourage a young athlete from long term participation in an activity that can be both fun and rewarding.

Mode of training

Several different types of exercises have been used to perform resistance exercises in children. Some that have been used include free weights, weight machines, body weight exercises (ie, push-ups or pull-ups), rubber tubing, medicine balls, and plyometrics.

It is important to consider the varying abilities of the children that will be participating when choosing the type of exercise to include in a strength training program. Some children may not be able to exert enough strength to successfully perform certain body weight exercises, such as push-ups or pull-ups. The preadolescent athlete may not be big enough to perform certain movements on adult sized equipment. Child-sized weight machines are available, but they are often difficult to find and can be quite expensive to purchase. Simply adding some extra padding to adult size equipment may resolve this discrepancy.

Free weights may be a good option for children because they are inexpensive, widely available, and allow for more variability between loads than some adult sized weight machines. They do, however, require close supervision to avoid injury from improper use. When free weights are chosen as a strength training modality, the authors feel that barbells are safer for children than dumbbells. Barbells promote better form and do not lend themselves as easily to the swinging, bounding movements sometimes common to lifting with dumbbells.

Among the several strength training exercises that can be chosen to include in a strength training program, a focus should be made on including exercises that strengthen the "core" of a young athletes body (low back, abdomen, and hips) [9,11]. Examples of core strengthening exercises include sit-ups, back extensions, and exercises rotational exercises performed with a medicine ball [9,11]. Including core exercises in a strength training program can help an athlete avoid injuries by strengthening the areas most commonly injured in youth sports [8].

Among the different types of exercises to include in a strength training program are exercises that involve single joints and those that involve multiple joints. Single-joint exercises are those that target a specific muscle group. Examples of single-joint exercises include leg-extensions and bicep curls, where only a single joint is involved in the movement. Examples of multi-joint exercises include the squat (Fig. 1) and bench press. Although multi-joint exercises are technically more difficult to master, they provide additional benefit to the athlete by incorporating coordination, balance, and proprioception into the workout program. That having been said, great care and close supervision with double spotting should be used when

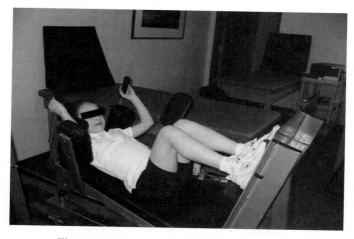

Fig. 1. Multijoint strength training with a machine.

children perform squats. If this is not possible, machine leg presses are preferable and safer.

Examples of exercises that can be incorporated in a youth strength training program include the leg press, leg extension, leg curls (hamstrings), bench press, bent-over rows (using bench press for support), lateral raises (elbows bent, arms raised to shoulder level), bicep curls, tricep extensions, back extension (avoid hyperextension), and abdominal curls [25].

Another common misconception is developing a program geared to develop strengths specific to a particular sport. Recent literature has shown better overall improvement in sports participation with the inclusion of a whole-body strength training program, compared with those whose strength training program was designed around a specific sport or movement [11].

Rate of progression

Progression during a strength training program can lead to improved strength gains and make it more fun, as an athlete sees himself or herself set and reach goals. Work-out cards or journals can be very useful in helping children keep track of the exercises they are performing, the amount of weight they last used, and the number of sets and repetitions that they performed during the last work-out session. An additional benefit of using workout cards is that it helps children avoid competition with their peers by turning their focus to self-improvement.

The National Strength and Conditioning Association [18] recommends a gradual increase in resistance as an athlete's strength improves [10]. When a child is able to perform more than 10 to 12 repetitions with a given load, adding weight can help the athlete increase their strength. A 5% to 10% increase in overall load is appropriate for most children. This usually corresponds to a two to five pound weight increase [11].

Maintaining training induced gains and detraining

Because the amount of time an athlete spends strength training may fluctuate throughout the year, it is important to know how often an athlete needs to strength train to maintain the strength he or she has made. Some of the reasons for decreased participation may include time restrictions while they are participating in their sports season, scheduling conflicts, decreased motivation, or injury rehabilitation.

Sewall and Micheli [2] demonstrated the effect detraining has on strength gains in children. Prepubescent children (ages 10–11) initially weight trained using child-sized weight machines for 9 weeks, resulting in a mean strength increase of 42.9%. Following 9 weeks with no strength training, the participants were tested again, showing a decrease of 27.6%.

Faigenbaum and colleagues [21] similarly showed the effects detraining has on strength gains achieved during an initial strength training period. Children, ages 7 to 12, initially participated in an 8-week strength training program. Significant strength gains were documented, including a 53.5% strength gain in leg extension and a 41.1% increase in bench press strength, compared with a strength gain of only 7.9% in a control group. The experimental group then stopped strength training. After 8 weeks of detraining, the experimental group lost 19.3% of the upper body and 28.1% of the lower body strength they had gained during the initial strength training period.

Developing a program

Similar to participation in any other exercise requiring physical exertion, a preparticipation physical should be performed before beginning a strength training program. When developing a strength training program (Table 1) for children, it is important to consider the participant's previous strength training experience, program goals, and their previous and current sports involvement [22]. A training program should also vary in volume and intensity throughout the training year to avoid overtraining when the athlete's activity increases during their sports season [9]. For most children, limiting competition and training to a maximum of 18 to 20 hours per week is recommended, while very satisfactory levels of fitness and sports competence can be attained with as little as 10 to 12 hours per week [11].

A program should start with a 5 to 10 minute warm-up period consisting of stretching, low-intensity aerobics, and one to two light sets of resistance exercises [18]. Organizing the workout session with exercises for the larger muscle groups (ie, squat) being performed before those for the smaller muscle groups has been shown to work well for adults and is reasonable in children as well [11]. One to three sets of 13 to 15 repetitions of a variety of

Table 1
Sample workout program for an adolescent athlete

Sample workout for young athlete	
Warm-up: 5–10 minutes (low intensity aerobics, stretching, 1–2 sets of light resistance exercises)	
2–3 sets of 13–15 repetitions of the following exercises, 2–3 times per week	
Exercise	Primary muscle involved
Bench press	Pectoralis major
Bent-over rows	Latissimus dorsi
Lateral raises	Deltoid
Bicep curls	Biceps brachii
Tricep extensions	Triceps
Machine leg presses	Quadriceps and hamstrings
Calf raises	Gastrocnemius/soleus
Abdominal crunches	Rectus abdominus

exercises should be performed on two to three nonconsecutive days per week. Resistance should be increased gradually (5%–10%) as strength increases. Varying the workout program can make strength training fun and keep participants interested, which is particularly important in a child's strength training program.

Instructors can also be a great encouragement for children, in addition to helping them focus on self-improvement rather than competition with peers. One instructor per ten children is an ideal ratio, although additional supervision may be necessary if participants are learning new exercises or strength training for the first time [9]. Some of the benefits of having a trained instructor present include maintaining a safe training environment, teaching children correct technique, proper breathing, and safe body mechanics. Professional certification is available through the National Strength and Conditioning Association [10].

Summary

Developing a strength training program for a preadolescent athlete that is both safe and effective involves the consideration of many variables. Some of these include: the age a child should begin strength training, the number of sets and repetitions an athlete should perform, how long to rest between sets, and how many times an athlete should exercise per week. While some of these variables have yet to be studied in the preadolescent athlete, knowledge of the current literature will help a coach or parent create a program for the child athlete that will help them be successful and avoid injury.

It is also important to remember that strength is only one component of overall fitness—both health related and sports specific. Appropriate attention must also be directed to flexibility and cardiovascular fitness, as well as on proper nutrition, when preparing a child athlete for safe and successful sports participation.

References

[1] Micheli L. Strength training in the young athlete. In: Brown E, Branta C, editors. Competitive sports for children and youth. Champaign (IL): Human Kinetics; 1988. p. 99–105.

[2] Sewall L, Micheli L. Strength training in children. J Pediatr Orthop 1986;6:143–6.

[3] Ramsay J, Blimkie C, Smith K, et al. Strength training effects in prepubescent boys. Med Sci Sports Exerc 1990;22:605–14.

[4] Faigenbaum A, Westcott W, Loud R, et al. The effects of different resistance training protocols on muscular strength and endurance development in children. Pediatrics 1999;104: 1–7.

[5] Falk B, Tenenbaum G. The effectiveness of resistance training in children: a meta-analysis. Sports Med 1996;22:176–86.

[6] Weltman A, Janney C, Rians C, et al. The effects of hydraulic-resistance strength training on prepubertal males. Med Sci Sports Exerc 1986;18:629–38.

[7] Outerbridge A, Micheli L. Overuse injuries in the young athlete. Clin Sports Med 1995;14: 503–16.

[8] Risser W, Risser J, Preston D. Weight training injuries in adolescents. Am J Dis Child 1990; 144:1015–7.

[9] Faigenbaum A, Risser J. Strength training for children and adolescents. Clin Sports Med 2000;19(4):593–619.

[10] Faigenbaum A, Kraemer W, Cahill B, et al. Youth resistance training: position statement paper and literature review. Strength Conditioning 1996;18(6):62–75.

[11] Faigenbaum A, Micheli L. Preseason conditioning for the preadolescent athlete. Pediatr Ann 2000;29(3):156–61.

[12] Bertelloni S, Ruggeri S, Baroncelli G. Effects of sports training in adolescence on growth, puberty and bone health. Gynecol Endocrinol 2006;22(11):605–12.

[13] Smith A, Andrish J, Micheli L. The prevention of sports injuries of children and adolescents. Med Sci Sports Exerc 1993;25(Suppl 8):1–7.

[14] Henja W, Roseberg A, Buturusis D, et al. The prevention of sports injuries in high school students through strength training. National Strength and Conditioning Assoc J 1982;4: 28–31.

[15] Faigenbaum A, Micheli L. Current Comment on Youth Strength Training. Indianapolis: American College of Sports Medicine; 1998.

[16] Hakkinen K, Mero A, Kauhanen H. Specificity of endurance, sprint and strength training on physical performance capacity in young athletes. J Sports Med Phys Fitness 1989;29(1): 27–35.

[17] Guy J, Micheli L. Strength training for children and adolescents. J Am Acad Orthop Surg 2001;9:29–36.

[18] Vrijens F. Muscle strength development in the pre- and post-pubescent age. Medicine and Sport 1978;11:152–8.

[19] American Academy of Pediatrics. Weight training and weight lifting: information for the pediatrician. Phys Sportsmed 1983;11:157–61.

[20] Falk B, Mor G. The effects of resistance and martial arts training in 6–8 year old boys. Pediatr Exerc Sci 1996;8:48–56.

[21] Faigenbaum A, Wescott W, Micheli L. The effects of strength training and detraining in children. Journal of Strength Training and Conditioning Research 1996;10:109–14.

[22] Faigenbaum A, Milliken L, Loud R, et al. Comparison of 1 and 2 days per week of strength training in children. Res Q Exerc Sport 2002;73(4):416–24.

[23] Faigenbaum A, Zaichkowsky L, Westcott W, et al. The effects of a twice per week strength training program on children. Pediatr Exerc Sci 1993;5:339–46.

[24] Faigenbaum A, Loud R, O'Connell J, et al. Effects of different resistance training protocols on upper-body strength and endurance development in children. J Strength Cond Res 2001; 15(4):459–65.

[25] Gyr B. Strength Training in Children and Adolescents. In: Delee J, Drez D, editors. Drez's Orthopaedic sports medicine: principles and practice, 2nd edition, vol. 1. Philadelphia: Saunders; 2003. p. 730–5.

[26] Faigenbaum A, Westcott W, Long C, et al. Relationship between repetitions and selected percentages of the one repetition maximum in healthy children. Pediatr Phys Ther 1998; 10:110–3.

[27] DeLorme T. Restoration of muscle power by heavy-resistance exercises. J Bone Joint Surg 1945;27:645–67.

[28] Rhea M, Alvar B, Ball S, et al. Three sets of weight training superior to 1 set with equal intensity for eliciting strength. J Strength Cond Res 2002;16(4):525–9.

[29] Wolfe B, LeMura L, Cole P. Quantitative analysis of single- vs. multiple-set programs in resistance training. J Strength Cond Res 2004;18(1):35–47.

[30] Schlumberger A, Stec J, Schmidtbleicher D. Single- vs multiple-set strength training in women. J Strength Cond Res 2001;15(3):284–9.

[31] Richmond S, Godard M. The effects of varied rest periods between sets to failure using the bench press in recreationally trained men. J Strength Cond Res 2004;18(4):846–9.

[32] Hill-Haas S, Bishop D, Dawson B. Effects of rest interval during high-repetition resistance training on strength, aerobic fitness, and repeated-sprint ability. J Sports Sci 2007;25(6): 619–28.
[33] Willardson J, Burkett L. The effects of rest interval length on bench press performance with heavy vs light loads. J Strength Cond Res 2006;20(2):396–9.
[34] Willardson J, Burkett L. A comparison of 3 different rest intervals on the exercise volume completed during a workout. J Strength Cond Res 2005;19(1):23–6.

ELSEVIER
SAUNDERS

Phys Med Rehabil Clin N Am
19 (2008) 247–269

PHYSICAL MEDICINE
AND REHABILITATION
CLINICS OF
NORTH AMERICA

Adolescent Sports Concussion

Cara Camiolo Reddy, MD[a,*],
Michael W. Collins, PhD[b], Gerald A. Gioia, PhD[c,d]

[a]Department of Physical Medicine and Rehabilitation, University of Pittsburgh Medical
Center, 3471 Fifth Avenue, LKB Suite 201, Pittsburgh, PA 15213, USA
[b]Department of Orthopaedic Surgery, University of Pittsburgh Medical Center,
3200 South Water Street, Pittsburgh, PA 15203, USA
[c]Department of Pediatrics, George Washington University School of Medicine and Children's
National Medical Center, 14801 Physician's Lane, Suite 173, Rockville, MD 20850, USA
[d]Department of Psychiatry, George Washington University School of Medicine and Children's
National Medical Center, 14801 Physician's Lane, Suite 173, Rockville, MD 20850, USA

Approximately 2 million sports and recreation concussive injuries occur per year in the United States [1]. Due to inconsistent data reporting, this is likely an underestimation of actual cases. The field of concussion management has evolved rapidly over the last 10 years, and with these advances comes new understanding of the significant symptomatic and cognitive impairments of concussion. These sequelae are more fully realized and may last longer than previously thought. Data have emerged regarding pathophysiology of concussion, risk factors, outcome, effects of repetitive injury, subtypes of concussive injury, and treatment protocols. This evidence calls for more conservative management of concussion, particularly in younger athletes, and demonstrates the shortcomings of concussion guidelines.

The practice of concussion management is moving from a general grading or guideline system toward individualized management based on scientific evidence of varied symptom presentations and recovery courses. Management protocols currently individualize assessment with the use of neurocognitive testing and comprehensive symptom evaluation. These evidence-based paradigms are emerging as the standard of care for management of concussion and return-to-play decisions.

Definition

Over the years, various academic organizations have proposed specific definitions of concussion; however, any definition of concussion has yet to

---

* Corresponding author.
  E-mail address: camioloce1@upmc.edu (C.C. Reddy).

1047-9651/08/$ - see front matter © 2008 Elsevier Inc. All rights reserved.
doi:10.1016/j.pmr.2007.12.002

be accepted universally. This lack of consensus becomes especially problematic when evaluating athletes in the field and determining whether an athlete has sustained a concussion or is experiencing pre-existing or unrelated symptoms. The Committee on Head Injury Nomenclature of Neurological Surgeons [2] and the American Academy of Neurology (AAN) [3] have proposed two such definitions that have been widely cited. The Committee on Head Injury Nomenclature of Neurological Surgeons defined concussion as "a clinical syndrome characterized by the immediate and transient post-traumatic impairment of neural function such as alteration of consciousness, disturbance of vision or equilibrium, etc., due to brain stem dysfunction." The American Academy of Neurology defined concussion as "any trauma induced alteration in mental status that may or may not include a loss of consciousness."

Most recently, the Centers for Disease Control and Prevention proposed a comprehensive definition of concussion. This definition aims to educate clinicians of the individualized nature of the injury, identifying key concepts that allow for a flexible approach to diagnosing and managing the injury. The Centers for Disease Control and Prevention definition reads [4]:

> "A mild traumatic brain injury (mTBI) or concussion is defined as a complex pathophysiologic process affecting the brain, induced by traumatic biomechanical forces secondary to direct or indirect forces to the head. MTBI is caused by a jolt to the head or body that disrupts the function of the brain. This disturbance of brain function is typically associated with normal structural neuroimaging findings (ie, CT scan, MRI). MTBI results in a constellation of physical, cognitive, emotional and or sleep-related symptoms that may or may not involve a loss of consciousness (LOC). Duration of symptoms is highly variable and may last from several minutes to days, weeks, months, or longer in some cases."

Pathophysiology

Recent work by Giza [5] and Hovda and colleagues [6] in animal models has led to insight regarding the pathophysiology of mild traumatic brain injury (TBI). Their findings suggested that concussion is a metabolic brain injury, rather than structural, with acute, posttraumatic changes occurring in intracellular and extracellular environments. These changes result from excitatory amino acid–induced ionic shifts associated with increased Na/K ATPase activation and resultant hyperglycolysis [7]. This process is accompanied by a decrease in cerebral blood flow that is not well understood, although it may be secondary to accumulation of endothelial calcium, which is thought to cause widespread cerebral neurovascular constriction. The resulting "metabolic mismatch" between energy demand and energy supply has been postulated to propagate a cellular vulnerability that is particularly susceptible to even minor changes in cerebral blood flow, increases in intracranial pressure, and apnea. Such metabolic dysfunction is theoretically linked to second impact syndrome and may form the basis for the less severe—although potentially incapacitating—postconcussion syndrome [8].

Animal models have indicated that this dysfunction can last up to 2 weeks or theoretically longer in the human model and can occur in athletes with normal Glasgow coma scores [5]. Traditional neurodiagnostic techniques (eg, CT scan, MRI, neurologic examination) are almost invariably normal after concussive insult [9]. It should be stressed, however, that these techniques are invaluable in ruling out more serious pathology (eg, cerebral bleeding and skull fracture) that may occur with head trauma.

On-field management

The diagnosis of cerebral concussion can be difficult, even in ideal circumstances. Athletes may have had neither direct trauma to the head nor loss of consciousness (LOC). Athletes may be unaware that they have been injured immediately after the injury and may not show any obvious signs of concussion, such as clumsiness, gross confusion, or obvious amnesia. To complicate this situation, athletes at all levels of competition may minimize or hide symptoms in an attempt to prevent their removal from the game, which creates the potential for exacerbation of the injury. Appropriate acute care and management of athletes with concussion begin with a detailed and accurate assessment of the nature and severity of the injury. As with any serious injury, the first priority is always to evaluate an athlete's level of consciousness and airway, breathing, and circulation.

Sideline presentation of symptoms may vary widely from athlete to athlete, depending on the biomechanical forces involved, severity of injury, affected brain areas, and an athlete's prior history of injury. Given the subtleties and variation in the presentation of a concussive injury, a thorough assessment of all signs and symptoms is crucial in making an accurate diagnosis of concussion. After a concussion, athletes may present with as few as one symptom or a constellation of many postconcussion symptoms, any and all of which are important from a diagnostic and management standpoint (Table 1).

Key acute signs

Loss of consciousness

Upon ruling out more severe injury, the acute evaluation continues with assessment of concussion. Several possible tools are available to guide physicians in their evaluation, including the acute concussion evaluation and the materials in the Centers for Disease Control and Prevention's toolkit for physicians, "Heads Up: Brain Injury in Your Practice" [4]. First, a clinician should establish the presence of any LOC. By definition, LOC represents

Table 1
Signs and symptoms of sports concussion

Signs observed by staff	Symptoms reported by athlete
Appears to be dazed or stunned	Headache
Is confused about assignment	Nausea
Forgets plays	Balance problems or dizziness
Is unsure of game, score, or opponent	Double or fuzzy/blurry vision
Moves clumsily	Sensitivity to light or noise
Answers questions slowly	Feeling sluggish or slowed down
Loses consciousness	Feeling "foggy" or groggy
Shows behavior or personality change	Concentration or memory problems
Forgets events before play (retrograde)	Change in sleep pattern (appears later)
Forgets events after hit (posttraumatic)	Feeling fatigued

a state of brief coma in which the eyes are typically closed and the athlete is unresponsive to external stimuli. The athlete who has a concussion is infrequently rendered unconscious, with studies indicating that 4% to 10% of sports-related concussions result in LOC [10,11]. Prolonged LOC (>1–2 min) in sports-related concussion is much less frequent [12], and athletes with LOC are typically unresponsive for only a brief period. Any athlete with documented LOC should be managed conservatively, and return to play is contraindicated.

Confusion

Confusion or disorientation, by definition, represents impaired awareness and orientation to surroundings, although memory systems are not directly affected. Confusion is often manifested by an athlete appearing stunned, dazed, or glassy-eyed on the sideline. Confusion is frequently revealed in athletes having difficulty with appropriate play calling, answering questions slowly or inappropriately, or repeating oneself during evaluation. Teammates are often the first to recognize that an athlete has been injured given the level of disorientation and difficulty in maintaining the flow of the game. Upon direct evaluation by the physician or athletic trainer, the athlete may be slow to respond. To assess properly the presence of confusion, simple orientation questions can be asked to the athlete (eg, name, current stadium, city, opposing team, current month and day) (Box 1).

Retrograde and anterograde amnesia

A careful evaluation of amnesia is of paramount importance in the athlete who has a concussion. Amnesia may be associated with loss of memory for events preceding or after injury. Specifically, posttraumatic amnesia or anterograde amnesia (synonymous terms) is typically represented by the length of time between trauma and the point at which the individual regains normal continuous memory functioning. As outlined in Box 1, on-field anterograde amnesia may be assessed through immediate and delayed (eg, 0, 5,

---

Box 1. University of Pittsburgh Medical Center's sideline concussion card: acute mental status testing

On-field cognitive testing
Orientation (ask the athlete the following questions)
   What stadium is this?
   What city is this?
   Who is the opposing team?
   What month is it?
   What day is it?
Posttraumatic amnesia (ask the athlete to repeat the following
   words): girl, dog, green
Retrograde amnesia (ask the athlete the following questions)
   What happened in the prior quarter or half?
   What do you remember just before the hit?
   What was the score of the game before the hit?
   Do you remember the hit?
Concentration (ask the athlete to do the following)
   Repeat the days of the week backward, starting with today
   Repeat these numbers backward: 63, 419
Word list memory
   Ask the athlete to repeat the three words from earlier
   (girl, dog, green)

---

15 minutes) memory for three words (eg, girl, dog, green). It should be noted that confusion and anterograde amnesia are not mutually exclusive and may be hard to dissociate. To help clarify this issue, anterograde amnesia represents a loss in memory from the point of injury until the return of a full, ongoing memory process. Confusion in and of it itself is not associated with memory loss. These two markers of injury may be assessed properly once the athlete's confusion is clear and lucid mental status returns. At that point, simply ask the athlete to recall the specific events that occurred immediately subsequent to trauma (eg, memory of returning to sideline, memory for subsequent plays, memory of later parts of contest). Any failure to recall these events properly indicates anterograde amnesia. Any presence of amnesia, even in seconds, has been found to be highly predictive of postinjury neurocognitive and symptom deficit [12].

Retrograde amnesia, although given less focus in the literature, is also an important injury severity marker of concussion. Retrograde amnesia is defined as the inability to recall events that occurred during the period immediately preceding trauma. To assess on-field retrograde amnesia properly, athletes may be asked questions pertaining to details occurring just before the trauma that caused the concussion. As Box 1 highlights, asking athletes to recall details of the injury is a good starting point. From there, asking athletes to recall the score of the game before the hit, events that occurred in the plays preceding the injury, and events that occurred in the first quarter or earlier in practice is a practical assessment strategy. It should be noted that the length of retrograde amnesia typically "shrinks" over time. For example, as recovery occurs, the length of retrograde amnesia may contract from hours to several minutes or even seconds, although by definition, a permanent loss of memory preceding injury occurs. Once again, even seconds of retrograde amnesia may be considered pathognomonic and predictive of outcome.

Symptoms

A thorough assessment of symptoms is critically important in an appropriate evaluation of a concussion. Four classes of symptoms should be assessed (ie, somatic, cognitive, emotional, sleep), although certain symptoms are more prevalent or may be manifested in the earlier or later stages of the injury (Fig. 1). For obvious reasons, sleep-related symptoms are not present on the day of the injury; however, they may be a significant issue after the first night's sleep. The following sections highlight several key symptoms often seen early in the injury.

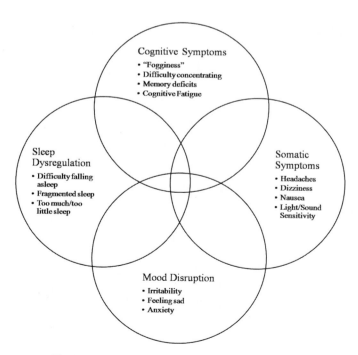

Fig. 1. Symptom clusters of postconcussion syndrome.

Headaches (somatic)

Headaches are the most commonly reported symptom of concussion and have been reported in up to 70% of athletes who have concussion [13]. Assessment of postconcussion headache is often complicated by the presence of musculoskeletal or myofascial pain–driven headaches that result from whiplash injury, cognitive fatigue headaches (discussed later), or premorbid headache and migraine exacerbation. Headaches caused by concussion may not develop immediately after injury and often do not develop until many hours after injury. Postconcussion headache is worsened with physical exertion; if the athlete complains of worsening headache during exertional testing or return to play, conservative management is indicated. The quality and location of the postconcussion headache seem to be consistent across the duration of recovery and infrequently change in location or character, with the exception of headaches influenced by myofascial pain generators, which can evolve during treatment. Although headache after a concussion does not necessarily constitute a medical emergency, a severe or progressively severe headache, particularly when accompanied by vomiting or rapidly declining mental status, may signal a life-threatening situation and should prompt immediate transport to hospital and CT scan of the brain.

Because of the prevalence of headache in individuals who have concussion, the relationship of headache to outcome was examined recently. One study examined high school athletes who had concussion and reported headache at approximately 1 week after injury versus athletes who did not report headache at that postinjury assessment. Results indicated that athletes with headaches performed significantly worse on measures of reaction time and memory, reported significantly more symptoms on the Post-Concussion Symptoms Scale, and were more likely to have experienced on-field anterograde amnesia than were athletes who did not report headaches [13]. Another recent project that examined headache type and outcome from concussion emphasized the importance of properly characterizing the postconcussion headache. Athletes who reported posttraumatic headaches with migrainous features (eg, nausea, vomiting, photophobia, or phonophobia) demonstrated more pronounced cognitive deficits at postinjury testing than athletes with no headaches or athletes with headaches without migrainous features [14].

Balance (somatic)

The vestibular system is susceptible to injury with trauma of the head and neck and can occur in the absence of skull base fractures or intracranial pathology [15]. Benign paroxysmal positional vertigo, labyrinthine concussion, perilymphatic fistulae, central vestibular disorders, endolymphatic hydrops, and cervicogenic vertigo have been reported after TBI, and several studies have documented balance deficits in athletes who have concussion [15–18].

Vestibular therapy, including repositioning techniques for benign paroxysmal positional vertigo, has been successful in managing these symptoms [19], and referral to a trained vestibular therapist is warranted in athletes with debilitating or ongoing vestibular symptoms.

Mental "fogginess" (cognitive)

Another frequently reported symptom gaining recent research attention is a reported sensation of feeling "foggy" after concussion [20]. Such data have suggested that the presence of "fogginess" after injury may be associated with a more severe course and protracted recovery. High school athletes who endorsed feeling "foggy" on a symptoms inventory were compared with concussed athletes who did not endorse a sense of "fogginess." Results indicated that the group that felt foggy demonstrated significantly slower reaction times, attenuated memory performance, and slower processing speed via computerized neurocognitive testing. Athletes who felt foggy also endorsed a significantly higher number of other postconcussion symptoms when compared with the group who did not endorse fogginess.

Mood disturbances (emotional)

Changes in mood are another commonly reported or observed symptom after TBI. Most often, athletes report increased irritability or having a "shorter fuse." Other emotional changes may occur, however, such as sadness, depression, nervousness, and anxiety. Affect may be described by the athlete or parent as flattened or labile. Emotional changes may be brief (eg, a linebacker bursts into tears for 30 seconds on the sideline) or may be prolonged in the case of a more significant injury (athlete reports persistent depression).

Neurocognitive assessment

The most significant advancement in the field is the development and clinical implementation of neurocognitive testing programs that allow for a reliable and valid approach to quantifying major manifestations of the injury, tracking athletes in terms of recovery, and providing a dependent variable to research individual factors in recovery effectively [21,22]. Neurocognitive testing has contributed to the development of a more individualized and data-driven approach to concussion management. Because concussion is a "functional" rather than "structural" brain injury, neurocognitive testing recently was deemed the cornerstone of proper concussion management through the implementation of baseline testing (preseason/preinjury) and subsequent postinjury evaluations conducted until recovery is complete [23].

During the initial stages of recovery from sports concussion, computer-based neurocognitive testing procedures have several advantages and relatively few disadvantages when compared with more traditional (ie, "paper-and-pencil" tests) neurocognitive testing procedures. First, the use of computers allows for the evaluation of large numbers of student athletes with minimal manpower. This technology promotes the baseline assessment of an entire athletic team within a reasonable time period using minimal human resources. Second, data acquired through testing can be stored easily in a specific computer or computer network and can be accessed at a later date (eg, after injury). Not only does computerized testing promote the efficient clinical evaluation of the athlete but it also greatly expands the possibilities for research. Third, the use of the computer promotes more accurate measurement of cognitive processes, such as reaction time and information processing speed. Computerized assessment allows for the evaluation of response times that are accurate to 0.01 seconds, whereas traditional testing only allows for accuracy up to 1 to 2 seconds. Fourth, the use of the computer allows for the randomization of test stimuli that may help to improve the reliability of data across multiple administration periods, which minimizes the "practice effects" that naturally occur with multiple exposures to the stimuli. Finally, computer-based approaches allow for the rapid dissemination of clinical information to sports medicine clinicians.

In summary, many benefits are derived from a computer-based approach insofar as the technology has appropriate sensitivity, reliability, and validity to measure the subtle aspects of concussive injury. It should be noted that more comprehensive neurocognitive testing may be indicated in the postacute management of injury and for athletes who exhibit protracted and complicated recoveries. Some clinicians use a "hybrid" approach of complementary computerized and paper-and-pencil test batteries to delineate an athlete's status.

A potential disadvantage of computer-based neurocognitive testing involves its inappropriate use as a "stand-alone" diagnostic instrument. This approach fails to recognize the complexity of the injury and may not incorporate other pertinent data, such as a detailed clinical interview, overall symptom presentation, medical/concussion history, and the results of other diagnostic studies (eg, balance testing, vestibular assessment).

Currently, several computer-based management approaches have been developed and validated to help determine management and return-to-play issues after concussive injury. Specifically, four computer-based models have been detailed in the scientific literature, including ImPACT (Immediate Post-Concussion Assessment and Cognitive Testing), CogState, Headminders, and ANAM (Automated Neurocognitive Assessment Matrices). Each of these test batteries has examined important aspects of reliability and validity in their approach to measuring concussive injury. Specific computerized test batteries have published additional data examining sensitivity/specificity of their test battery and the "added value" of their assessment tool when compared with the assessment of symptoms in isolation [24–26].

Neurocognitive deficits that result from concussion have been documented in many studies, and cognitive testing seems to be a highly valuable tool in documenting impairment or incomplete recovery from concussive injury. Neurocognitive deficits associated with concussion also have been documented in studies of collegiate football players, high school football players, amateur soccer players, and samples of athletes who have concussion across multiple sports. Neurocognitive evaluation is a sensitive tool that may be used to assess the often subtle and potentially debilitating effects of concussive injury. Neurocognitive test data seem to provide objective, quantifiable, and individualized standards to better determine safe return to participation and overall management of the athlete who has concussion and should be considered a critical factor in concussion management.

Treatment paradigm

There are no curative medical treatments for concussion, and clinical observation suggestions that exertion—both physical and cognitive—can delay recovery. This finding underscores the importance of early identification, evaluation, and management of a concussion and the resultant symptoms and prevention of additional injury or exacerbation of a current injury through early return to physical exertion or early return to play. In the initial days after injury, athletes should be instructed on the benefits of proper sleep hygiene, physical rest, and cognitive rest.

Based on published data, approximately 80% of athletes spontaneously recover within 3 weeks of trauma, with the remaining 20% having a "protracted" recovery [27,28]. Given the strong relationship between exertion and recovery, there has been interest in creating specific concussion rehabilitation protocols that focus on graded exertional protocols from a physical and cognitive perspective. Research is forthcoming regarding this issue.

The diagnosis of postconcussion syndrome is controversial in the medical community, because the symptoms associated with concussion can appear vague and be mistaken for other clinical issues. Despite this debate, distinct symptom clusters and neurocognitive deficits after concussion have been identified. Specific treatment recommendations also may include pharmacologic interventions based on symptom clusters that the athlete may be experiencing. From a treatment standpoint, it has been the philosophy of these authors to avoid pharmacologic intervention until the athlete is at 3 weeks or longer into recovery and there is functional disability as it relates to the experienced symptoms (eg, difficulties in school, severe symptoms) (Fig. 1).

A detailed history is imperative for evaluation and treatment of concussion, including mechanism of injury, location of the impact, length of LOC (if present), presence of retrograde or anterograde amnesia, initial symptoms, and treatment. A comprehensive review of ongoing symptoms should be undertaken. Symptoms consistent with concussion fall into four categories: cognitive, somatic, emotional, and sleep disturbance.

Cognitive

Neurocognitive testing has provided objective data illustrating the multitude of cognitive derangements after concussion. Clinically, individuals may complain of feeling foggy, not being able to think quickly, or not being able to focus attention to complete everyday tasks. Students often complain of declining academic performance. Short-term memory deficits and prolonged reaction times are also apparent. There is clear evidence that the cognitive deficits after TBI improve with the addition of neurostimulant medications [29]. Most of these data involve the more severely brain injured populations; however, the improvements in neurocognitive testing are compelling. Anecdotally, substantial clinical improvement has been noted in individuals treated with methylphenidate, amantadine, or atomoxetine. (Please note that these are off-label uses for these medications.)

Somatic

Headaches are one of the most common symptoms after concussion. Getting specific information regarding the character of the headache is important, because posttraumatic headaches can be caused by multiple underlying causes, including musculoskeletal, vascular, neuropathic, and iatrogenic factors. A thorough history and physical examination help to narrow down these potential causes and help to dictate a treatment plan. Some varieties of posttraumatic headache have been found to be amenable to the same treatment guidelines available for primary headaches and migraines [30]. Prophylactic treatment with beta-blockers, calcium-channel blockers, and antidepressants can play a role. Infrequent posttraumatic migraines also may benefit from abortive medications in the triptan family. Musculoskeletal or tension headaches can be further identified by complaint of pain at the temples or tender spots and decreased neck range of motion on physical examination.

Of particular note, some individuals complain of headaches that occur only in the setting of "cognitive exertion." For example, athletes who have concussion may complain of headaches that occur and worsen with activities, including taking notes in class or taking tests. Often these individuals also endorse significant cognitive symptoms. These headaches are associated with symptoms of "feeling foggy" or difficulty concentrating. Such headaches have been dubbed by these authors as "cognitive-fatigue" headaches: those that occur in clear relationship with cognitive exertion. For this subtype of headache, treating the cognitive symptoms (rather than the headaches themselves) may prove to be more efficacious. Preliminary data suggest that neurostimulants may aid in headache management by improving the cognitive deficits that act as their trigger. Further research in this arena is warranted.

Emotional

Prolonged, unresolving cognitive and somatic symptoms may cause many individuals to become frustrated and anxious. Mood disorders, including depression, are frequently seen after TBI. These emotional disturbances may worsen perception of cognitive impairment or pain. Initiation of selective serotonin reuptake inhibitors has been shown to be particularly helpful and may have an added benefit of headache prevention.

Sleep disturbance

Disorders of sleep are also well documented after TBI [31]. Although individuals may initially complain of hypersomnia, several weeks after injury they often complain of difficulty falling asleep or staying asleep. Normal sleep-wake patterns can quickly become dysregulated. Proper sleep hygiene, including going to bed and waking at the same times daily, limiting caffeine intake, reducing daytime naps, and eliminating TV watching in bed, should be advocated. Medications such as trazodone, amitriptyline, or melatonin can be used to improve the quality and quantity of sleep. Benzodiazepines and nonbenzodiazepine hypnotics should be avoided because of their amnestic qualities and potential worsening of cognitive functioning.

Predictors of outcome after concussion

Two published studies examined on-field predictors of outcome after sports-related concussion. Collins and colleagues [12] investigated the relationship between on-field markers of concussion severity and postinjury neurocognitive performance and symptom presentation in a group of 78 high school and college athletes who had concussion. Data from this study revealed that the presence of amnesia was most predictive of postinjury difficulties at 3 days after injury. Athletes who demonstrated notable cognitive deficits and high degree of symptoms were more than ten times more likely to have exhibited any degree of retrograde amnesia after concussion when compared with athletes with no cognitive deficits and no reported symptoms at 3 days after injury. Similarly, athletes with cognitive deficits and high degree of symptoms were more than four times more likely to have exhibited any degree of anterograde amnesia.

Interestingly, LOC did not predict deficits after sports-related concussion. A second outcome study examined 47 athletes with concussion [32]. These researchers found that athletes who reported memory problems at follow-up examinations had significantly more symptoms in general, longer duration of symptoms, and significant decreases on neurocognitive test performance. Data from these two studies directly contradict existing grading systems of concussion, which all delineate severity of injury and length of time until return to play on the LOC construct. The outlined data suggest that amnesia, particularly retrograde amnesia, may be much more predictive in this regard.

A growing body of evidence suggests that there may be cumulative detrimental effects of multiple concussions. This effect has been associated with the neurocognitive impairment and neurologic abnormalities that primarily have been documented among boxers [33,34]. Matser and colleagues [35] also suggested that cumulative long-term consequences of repetitive blows to the head are being seen in professional soccer players. Lately, however, this topic has been of rising concern among other athletic populations, and the sequelae of multiple concussions in high school and collegiate athletes have been investigated [36,37].

High school and collegiate athletes who suffer three or more concussions seem to be more vulnerable to subsequent injury than athletes with no history of injury [38]. In a study of almost 400 college football players, Collins and colleagues [39] revealed long-term subtle neurocognitive deficits in athletes who suffered two or more concussions. Results indicated that high school athletes with a history of three previous concussions were more than nine times more likely than athletes without history of previous concussions to exhibit three or four on-field markers of injury (eg, LOC, amnesia, confusion) with a subsequent concussion. Guskiewicz and colleagues [37] examined repeated concussion in collegiate football players and found an association between self-reported history of previous concussion and subsequent concussion. Players with a history of at least three concussions also were three times more likely than athletes without previous concussion history to sustain an additional injury. Having a history of one or two previous concussions also elevated concussion risk. This study demonstrated that sustaining multiple concussions places high school athletes at greater risk for worse neurobehavioral outcomes.

Recent research has highlighted specific risk factors that seem to result in more protracted recovery in athletes who sustain concussive injury. Such factors include a pre-existing history of learning disability [39], younger age [40], and prior history of concussive injury, amnesia, and LOC [36,37]. Athletes who experienced posttraumatic migrainous symptoms exhibited longer recovery; the issue of migraine plays a significant role in recovery and perhaps treatment strategies [14]. The role of exertion on recovery from injury has been studied, and such data clearly indicate the need for moderation of physical and cognitive exertion during the acute stages of recovery [41].

Return to play

Concussion grading systems

During the past 30 years, more than 20 concussion management guidelines have been published with the intent of providing direction for sports medicine practitioners in making complex return-to-play decisions [42]. The authors of each of these guidelines also provided an accompanying grading scale designed to reflect and characterize the severity of the injury. Although these guidelines undoubtedly have resulted in improved care of athletes, these multiple directives created significant confusion and sparked almost continuous debate (Table 2).

Table 2
Concussion grading scales

Guideline	Grade 1	Grade 2	Grade 3
Cantu [43]	No LOC *and* post-traumatic amnesia lasts <30 min	LOC lasts longer than 5 minutes *or* posttraumatic amnesia lasts >30 min	LOC lasts >5 min *or* posttraumatic amnesia lasts >24 h
Colorado [44]	Confusion without amnesia *and* no LOC	Confusion with amnesia *and* no LOC	LOC of any duration
American Academy of Neurology [3]	Transient confusion without LOC, symptoms/mental status changes resolve in <5 min	Transient confusion without LOC, symptoms/mental status change lasts > 15 min	LOC of any duration
Cantu – revised [45]	No LOC *or* posttraumatic amnesia/symptoms lasting >30 min	LOC <1 min *or* posttraumatic amnesia >30 min and <24 h	LOC >1 min *or* posttraumatic amnesia >24 h *or* postconcussion symptoms >7 d

Cantu [43] originally proposed his grading scale and management guidelines based on clinical experience; however, he was careful to emphasize that these guidelines were intended to supplement rather than replace clinical judgment. The original guidelines allowed return to play the day of injury if the athlete were symptom free at rest and after physical exertion. For athletes who experienced any LOC (eg, grade 3 concussion), a restriction of contact for 1 month was recommended. Athletes who had suffered a grade 2 concussion were allowed to return to play in 2 weeks if asymptomatic for a period of 7 days.

The Colorado Guidelines, which were drafted under the auspices of the Colorado Medical Society [44], were published in 1991 after a high school athlete died as a result of second impact syndrome. These guidelines allowed for same-day return to play if symptoms cleared within 20 minutes of injury. For more severe injury (grade 3 concussion), immediate transport to a hospital for further evaluation was recommended. These guidelines were later revised under the sponsorship of the American Academy of Neurology [3], whose guidelines allowed return to competition the same day of injury if an athlete's signs and symptoms cleared within 15 minutes of injury. Grade 2 concussions were managed in a manner similar to the Colorado Guidelines, with return to competition within 1 week if asymptomatic.

More recently, Cantu [45] amended his guidelines to emphasize the duration of posttraumatic symptoms in grading the severity of the concussion and making return-to-play decisions. Grade 1 concussion was redefined by an absence of LOC and postconcussion signs or symptoms lasting less than 30 minutes. Same-day return to competition was allowed only if the athlete was completely asymptomatic after the injury.

New paradigms for concussion evaluation and management

Although the management guidelines reached their zenith of popularity during the 1980s and 1990s, in the late 1990s, sports medicine practitioners and organizations began to question the scientific basis of these guidelines. This trend prompted the American Orthopaedic Society for Sports Medicine to sponsor a workshop with the purpose of re-evaluating current guidelines and establishing practical alternatives [46]. Although their guidelines did not differ substantially from prior guidelines, it marked a new trend in concussion grading that moved away from the use of numeric grading systems for determination of return to play after concussion. The American Orthopaedic Society for Sports Medicine guidelines were also the first to stress more individualized management of injury rather than applying general standards and protocols.

Another important development in clinical concussion management took place in 2002 under the auspices of the Federation Internationale de Football Association in conjunction with the International Olympic Committee and the International Ice Hockey Federation. The organizers of this meeting assembled a group of physicians, neuropsychologists, and sports administrators in Vienna, Austria to continue to explore methods of reducing morbidity secondary to sports-related concussion. The deliberations that took place during this meeting led to the publication of a document that outlined recommendations for the diagnosis and management of concussion in sports [23,47]. One of the most important conclusions of this meeting was that none of the previously published concussion management guidelines was adequate to ensure proper management of every concussion. The group emphasized the implementation of postinjury neurocognitive testing as the "cornerstone" of proper postinjury management and return-to-play decision making.

The recognition of neurocognitive testing as a key element of the postconcussion evaluation process represented a particularly important development in the diagnosis and management of the athlete who has concussion. The use of baseline neurocognitive testing was specifically recommended whenever possible. A graduated return-to-play protocol also was emphasized. The specific recommendations of the International Conference on Concussion in Sport are presented in Box 2. The group specifically recommended that each step would, in most circumstances, be separated by 24 hours. Any recurrence of concussive symptoms should lead to the athlete dropping back to the previous level. In other words, if an athlete is asymptomatic at rest and develops a headache after light aerobic exercise, the athlete should return to complete rest. The Vienna group further recognized that conventional structural neuroimaging studies (eg, CT scan, MRI, and electroencephalogram) are typically unremarkable after concussive injury and should be used only when a structural lesion is suspected. The group further suggested that functional imaging techniques are in the early stages of development but may provide valuable information in the future.

Box 2. Vienna concussion conference: return-to-play recommendations [23]

Athletes should complete the following step-wise process before return to play following after concussion:
1. Removal from contest after concussion
2. No return to play in current game
3. Medical evaluation after injury
   a. Rule out more serious intracranial pathology
   b. Neurocognitive testing considered "cornerstone" of proper postinjury assessment
4. Step-wise return to play
   a. No activity and rest until asymptomatic
   b. Light aerobic exercise
   c. Sport-specific training
   d. Noncontact drills
   e. Full-contact drills
   f. Game play

From Aubry M, Cantu R, Dvorak J, et al. Summary and agreement statement of the first International Conference on Concussion in Sport, Vienna 2001. Clin J Sport Med 2002;12(1):6.

Propelled by these recommendations, data-driven protocols currently are available to help manage an athlete after sports concussion injury. Once an athlete who has concussion has been removed from a game, the sports medicine physician is faced with the often challenging decision of when the athlete is safely able to return to play. Making return-to-play decisions, whether on the field or during the postinjury management of injury, can be one of the most difficult decisions facing sports medicine practitioners and represents a dynamic process that involves the evaluation of factors such as the severity of the injury, the athlete's reported symptoms, and performance on neurocognitive testing. In addition to these variables that relate to clinical recovery, several other potential factors may play a role in the decision-making process. Since the advent of neurocognitive testing, prospective data are emerging that begin to shed light on individual factors that may play a role in the incidence, severity, and length of recovery regarding concussion.

Individual factors that influence return to play

Age

The aforementioned concussion guidelines assume identical return-to-play criteria for athletes regardless of age and do not include developmental considerations, which are likely important when managing concussion in adolescence. Based on these guidelines, it has traditionally been assumed that the speed of recovery is the same at all age groups and athletic levels. Recent research has begun to shed light on potential differential age-related responses to concussive injury.

Based on research done with more severe TBI, several theories do exist that might explain age-related differences into recovery from concussion. One such theory is that children may undergo more prolonged and diffuse cerebral swelling after TBI, which suggests that they may be at increased risk for secondary injury [48,49]. The immature brain may be up to 60 times more sensitive to glutamate, a neurotransmitter involved in the metabolic cascade after concussion [50]. These factors may lead to a longer recovery period and could increase the likelihood of permanent or severe neurologic deficit should reinjury occur during the recovery period.

Theoretically, this sensitivity may account for the fact that second impact syndrome has been found only in adolescent athletes [8]. Sustaining a second head injury during a period of increased vulnerability with unresolved metabolic dysfunction has been linked to second impact syndrome. Varying reports suggest that as many as 35 or more athletes in the past decade have succumbed to this syndrome. In all cases, athletes were reported to have sustained an initial concussive injury, returned to sports or other activities, and then sustained a second, typically milder, concussive injury. The second blow resulted in purported dysautoregulation, massive edema, uncal herniation, and coma, which was followed by death shortly after the blow. Morbidity is 100% in the case of second impact syndrome, whereas mortality is reported to occur in up to 50% of cases.

One published study directly examined recovery from concussion in college-aged versus high school–aged athletes [40]. Specifically, baseline and postconcussion neurocognitive functioning was measured in a sample of 53 athletes. Although the college sample had a greater prior incidence of concussion, high school athletes were found to take longer to recover during an in-study concussion. This study suggested more protracted recovery from concussion in high school athletes. Another recently published study revealed the apparent heightened vulnerability to concussion in high school athletes [51]. Specifically, the issue of "bell ringers" or mild concussions was examined in high school athletes aged 13 to 17 years. This study revealed that high school athletes with less than 15 minutes of on-field symptoms required at least 7 days before full neurocognitive and symptom recovery. This study and a follow-up analysis called into question the validity of the grading systems for management of mild concussion [52]. These findings suggested that all high school athletes diagnosed with concussion be removed from play during that contest.

Gender

Recent trends in sport participation have seen increased participation of girls and women. To date, little research has specifically examined gender differences in concussion. Most published literature has focused on nonathletic populations and rodents. A recent meta-analysis of eight studies and 20 outcome variables in mild TBI studies unrelated to sports revealed that across 85% of those variables, outcome was worse in women [53]. These findings have suggested that women with mild TBI are more likely to report sleep disturbances and headaches up to a year after injury, may be less likely than men to be employed or in school 1 year after mild head injury, and suffer a significant decrease in grade point average compared with controls. There were no similar findings for men. Even when controlling for other demographic, premorbid, and event-related factors, most research to date has shown that women have worse outcomes than men after mild TBI.

Although the gender-based sports concussion literature is limited, a few studies have emerged. Barnes and colleagues [54] retrospectively demonstrated that male elite soccer players suffered concussions of greater severity and were subject to a higher incidence of injury than female elite soccer players. A prospective study involving 15 National Collegiate Athletic Association men's and women's soccer teams over two seasons revealed similar incidence of concussion in men and women.

Although much of the available literature reveals poorer outcome among women who suffer from TBI, animal models suggest that female sex hormones actually may protect neurons in the brain after concussive injury [55–57]. Progesterone is thought to reduce cerebral edema and potentially facilitate cognitive recovery, whereas studies of estrogen influence have yielded mixed results. Studies have shown estrogen to play a protective role in male subjects while increasing mortality in female subjects [58,59]. Other research has demonstrated that estrogen can assist in maintaining normal cerebral blood flow and actually decrease mortality when administered acutely. All of the aforementioned research suggests that important gender differences may impact the incidence and severity of TBI. More research in this area is necessary to accurately delineate the implications of such differences.

Learning disability

Learning disability refers to a heterogeneous group of disorders revealed by difficulties in the acquisition and use of listening, speaking, writing, reading, reasoning, or mathematical abilities, which are traditionally diagnosed in early childhood. Presence of a learning disability has been linked to lower baseline cognitive performance within a large, multi-university sample of football players [39]. Football players who had learning disabilities and reported a history of multiple concussions demonstrated reduced overall cognitive functioning when compared with athletes with multiple concussions who did not have a learning disability and when compared with individuals with no concussion history who had a learning disability, which suggested a potential additive effect. Ascertaining an educational history as part of the comprehensive evaluation of athletes is important, because the presence of learning disability certainly has the potential to complicate the diagnosis of concussion and the return-to-play decision.

Current return-to-play guidelines

Prevailing standards of care require an athlete to satisfy three general conditions before returning to play [23,47]. First, the athlete must demonstrate that he or she is completely symptom free at rest. The athlete should complete a symptom inventory or symptom interview on the sideline and serially throughout recovery. Before progressing to any significant level of physical exertion, the athlete should report being completely asymptomatic at rest. If the athlete's report of asymptomatic status is suspected to be false, a careful discussion of the importance of reporting all symptoms should be initiated with the athlete. Such cases should be augmented with formal neurocognitive testing (Table 3).

Second, as an athlete demonstrates being asymptomatic at rest, he or she should begin a graduated return to physical and cognitive exertion before contact participation, because postconcussion symptoms may evolve with increased metabolic demands. International consensus recommendations have suggested a graduated exertional protocol (described earlier). Such

Table 3
The postconcussion symptom inventory

Symptom	None	Minor		Moderate		Severe	
Headache	0	1	2	3	4	5	6
Nausea	0	1	2	3	4	5	6
Vomiting	0	1	2	3	4	5	6
Balance problems	0	1	2	3	4	5	6
Dizziness	0	1	2	3	4	5	6
Fatigue	0	1	2	3	4	5	6
Trouble falling asleep	0	1	2	3	4	5	6
Sleeping more than usual	0	1	2	3	4	5	6
Sleeping less than usual	0	1	2	3	4	5	6
Drowsiness	0	1	2	3	4	5	6
Sensitivity to light	0	1	2	3	4	5	6
Sensitivity to noise	0	1	2	3	4	5	6
Irritability	0	1	2	3	4	5	6
Sadness	0	1	2	3	4	5	6
Nervousness	0	1	2	3	4	5	6
Feeling more emotional	0	1	2	3	4	5	6
Numbness or tingling	0	1	2	3	4	5	6
Feeling slowed down	0	1	2	3	4	5	6
Feeling mentally "foggy"	0	1	2	3	4	5	6
Difficulty concentrating	0	1	2	3	4	5	6
Difficulty remembering	0	1	2	3	4	5	6
Visual problems	0	1	2	3	4	5	6

From Lovell MR, Collins MW. Neuropsychological assessment of the college football player. J Head Trauma Rehabil 1998;13:9–26; with permission.

a protocol may involve the athlete successfully moving through the following exertional stages: (1) light aerobic exercise (eg, walking, stationary biking), (2) sport-specific training of moderate exertion (eg, ice skating in hockey, running in soccer), and (3) noncontact training drills of heavy exertion (eg, heavy weight training, sprints, all positional maneuvers. If the athlete's previously resolved postconcussion symptoms return at any point during the graded return to physical exertion, the athlete should return to the previous exertion level at which he or she was last asymptomatic. In addition to physical exertion, cognitive exertion should be monitored closely along with its overall relationship to symptoms. Physical and cognitive exertion may have different effects on symptoms, and athletes must meet resolution criteria in both realms before progressing further.

Third, there is increasing evidence and agreement that the athlete should demonstrate intact neurocognitive functioning before return to sport participation. Postinjury assessment in the form of neurocognitive testing also should be considered to help determine overall management and return-to-participation issues. Cognitive recovery is considered achieved when the athlete's performance either returns to baseline levels or, in the absence of baseline, is consistent with premorbid estimates of functioning when the test data are compared with normative values. Many practitioners prefer to complete acute and serial follow-up evaluations to gain insight into the extent and type of cognitive impairment created by the injury. Such data can help with prognosis [60], help to determine when the athlete may return to exertion, and may help to provide academic recommendations and accommodations.

Once the athlete has been cleared medically, is symptom free at rest and with physical exertion, and falls within expected levels on cognitive testing, he or she may return to full-contact training and then to competition. Such evidence-based parameters are becoming the "gold standard" for return to sport participation after concussion and are becoming widely implemented at all levels of sports participation. Considerations according to prior history of concussion and outcome from previous concussion and any suspected deception in the athlete's symptom reporting may influence return to participation and management directives further, which highlights the need for individualized concussion evaluation and management.

References

[1] Langlois JA, Rutland-Brown W, Wald M. The epidemiology and impact of traumatic brain injury: a brief overview. J Head Trauma Rehabil 2006;21(5):375–8.
[2] Congress of Neurological Surgeons. Committee on head injury nomenclature: glossary of head injury. Clin Neurosurg 1996;12:386–94.
[3] Quality Standards Subcommittee. American Academy of Neurology. Practice parameter: the management of concussion in sports. Neurology 1997;48:581–5.

[4] Centers for Disease Control and Prevention (CDC). National Center for Injury Prevention and Control. Heads up: brain injury in your practice. Atlanta (GA): Centers for Disease Control and Prevention; 2007. Available at: http://www.cdc.gov/ncipc/tbi/Physicians_Tool_Kit.htm. Accessed October 1, 2007.

[5] Giza CC, Hovda DA. The neurometabolic cascade of concussion. J Athl Train 2001;36: 228–35.

[6] Hovda DA, Prins M, Becker DP. Neurobiology of concussion. In: Lovell MR, et al, editors. Sports related concussion. St. Louis (MO): Quality Medical Publishing; 1999. p. 12–51.

[7] Bergschneider M, Hovda DA, Shalmon E. Cerebral hyperglycolysis following severe human traumatic brain injury: a positron emission tomography study. J Neurosurg 2003;86:241–51.

[8] Cantu RC, Voy R. Second impact syndrome: a risk in any contact sport. Physician and Medicine 1995;23:27–34.

[9] McAllister TW, Sparling MB, Flashman LA, et al. New developments in management of sports concussion: neuroimaging findings in mild traumatic brain injury. J Clin Exp Neuropsychol 2001;23(6):775–91.

[10] Guskiewicz KM, Weaver NL, Padua DA, et al. Epidemiology of concussion in collegiate and high school football players. Am J Sports Med 2000;28:1–8.

[11] Schulz MR, Marshall SW, Mueller FO, et al. Incidence and risk factors for concussion in high school athletes, North Carolina, 1996–1999. Am J Epidemiol 2004;160:937–44.

[12] Collins MW, Iverson GL, Lovell MR, et al. On-field predictors of neuropsychological and symptom deficit following sports-related concussion. Clin J Sport Med 2003;13:222–9.

[13] Collins MW, Field M, Lovell MR, et al. Relationship between post-concussion headache and neuropsychological test performance in high school athletes. Am J Sports Med 2003; 31:168–73.

[14] Mihalik J, Stump J, Collins MW, et al. Posttraumatic migraine characteristics in athletes following sports-related concussion. J Neurosurg 2005;102:850–5.

[15] Ernst A, Basta D, Seidle RO, et al. Management of posttraumatic vertigo. Otolaryngol Head Neck Surg 2005;132:554–8.

[16] Peterson CL, Ferrara MS, Mrazik M, et al. Evaluation of neuropsychological domain scores and postural stability following cerebral concussion in sports. Clin J Sport Med 2003;13: 230–7.

[17] McCrea M, Guskiewicz KM, Marshall SW, et al. Acute effects and recovery time following concussion in collegiate football players. JAMA 2003;290(19):2556–63.

[18] Guskiewicz KM, Perrin DH, Bansneder BM. Effect of mild head injury on postural stability in athletes. J Athl Train 1996;31:300–6.

[19] Parnes LS, Price-Jones RG. Particle repositioning manoeuver for BPPV. Ann Otol Rhinol Laryngol 1993;102:325–31.

[20] Iverson GL, Gaetz M, Lovell MR, et al. Relation between subjective fogginess and neuropsychological testing following concussion. J Int Neuropsychol Soc 2004;10(6):904–6.

[21] Echemendia RJ, Putukian M, Macklin ML. Neuropsychological test performance prior to and following sports-related mild traumatic brain injury. Clin J Sport Med 2001;11:23–31.

[22] Grindel SH, Lovell MR, Collins MW. The assessment of sports-related concussions: the evidence behind neuropsychological testing and management. Clin J Sport Med 2001;11: 134–43.

[23] Aubry M, Cantu R, Dvorak J, et al. Summary and agreement statement of the first International Conference on Concussion in Sport, Vienna 2001. Clin J Sport Med 2002;12(1):6–10.

[24] Schatz P, Pardini JE, Lovell MR, et al. Sensitivity and specificity of the impact test battery for concussion in athletes. Arch Clin Neuropsychol 2006;21:91–9.

[25] van Kampen D, Lovell MR, Collins MW, et al. The "value added" of neurocognitive testing in managing sports concussion. Am J Sports Med 2006;34(10):1630–5.

[26] Fazio V, Lovell MR, Pardini J, et al. The relationship between post-concussion symptoms and neurocognitive performance in concussed athletes. NeuroRehabilitation 2007;22(3): 207–16.

[27] Collins MW, Lovell MR, Iverson GL, et al. Examining concussion rates and return to play in high school football players wearing newer helmet technology: a three year prospective cohort study. Neurosurgery 2006;58(2):275–84.

[28] Yang CC, Tu YK, Hua MS, et al. The association between the postconcussion symptoms and clinical outcomes for patient with mild traumatic brain injury. J Trauma 2007;62(3): 657–63.

[29] Warden DL, Gordon B, McAllister TW, et al. Guidelines for the pharmacologic treatment of neurobehavioral sequelae of traumatic brain injury. J Neurotrauma 2006;23(10):1468–501.

[30] Lew HL, Lin PH, Fuh JL, et al. Characteristics and treatment of headache after traumatic brain injury: a focused review. Am J Phys Med Rehabil 2006;85(7):619–27.

[31] Clinchot D, Bogner JA, Mysiw JW, et al. Defining sleep disturbances after brain injury. Am J Phys Med Rehabil 1998;77:291–5.

[32] Erlanger D, Kaushik T, Cantu R, et al. Symptom-based assessment of the severity of concussion. J Neurosurg 2003;98:34–9.

[33] Jordan BD, Relkin NR, Ravdin LD. Apolipoprotein e4 associated with chronic traumatic brain injury in boxing. JAMA 1997;278:136–40.

[34] Roberts SW, Allsop B, Bruton C. The occult aftermath of boxing. J Neurol Neurosurg Psychiatry 1990;53:373–8.

[35] Matser E, Kessels A, Lezak M. Neuropsychological impairment in amateur soccer players. JAMA 1998;282:971–4.

[36] Collins MW, Lovell MR, Iverson GL, et al. Cumulative effects of concussion in high school athletes. Neurosurgery 2002;51:1175–81.

[37] Guskiewicz KM, McCrea M, Marshall SW, et al. Cumulative effects associated with recurrent concussion in collegiate football players: the NCAA concussion study. JAMA 2003; 290(19):2549–55.

[38] Iverson GL, Gaetz M, Lovell MR, et al. Cumulative effects of concussion in amateur athletes. Brain Inj 2004;18:433–43.

[39] Collins MW, Grindel SH, Lovell MR, et al. Relationship between concussion and neuropsychological performance in college football players. JAMA 1999;282:964–70.

[40] Field M, Collins MW, Lovell MR, et al. Does age play a role in recovery from sports-related concussion? A comparison of high school and collegiate athletes. J Pediatr 2003;142(5): 546–53.

[41] Majerske CW, Mihalik JP, Dianxu R, et al. Concussion in sports: the effect of post-concussive activity levels on symptoms and neurocognitive performance. J Athl Train, in press.

[42] Collins MW, Lovell MR, McKeag DB. Current issues in managing sports-related concussion. JAMA 1999;282(24):2283–5.

[43] Cantu RC. Cerebral concussion in sport: management and prevention. Sports Med 1992;14: 64–74.

[44] Kelly JP, Nichols JS, Filley CM. Concussion in sports: guidelines for the prevention of catastrophic outcome. JAMA 1991;266:2867–9.

[45] Cantu RC. Posttraumatic retrograde and anterograde amnesia: pathophysiology and implications in grading and safe return to play. J Athl Train 2001;36:244–8.

[46] Wojtys ED, Hovda D, Landry G, et al. Concussion in sports. Am J Sports Med 1999;27: 676–86.

[47] McCrory P, Johnston K, Meeuwisse W, et al. Summary and agreement statement of the second International Conference on Concussion in Sport, Prague 2004. Br J Sports Med 2005; 29:196–204.

[48] Pickles W. Acute general edema of the brain in children with head injuries. N Engl J Med 1950;242(16):607–11.

[49] Bruce DA, Alvai A, Bilaniuk L, et al. Diffuse cerebral swelling following head injuries in children: the syndrome of malignant brain edema. J Neurosurg 1981;54:170–8.

[50] McDonald JW, Johnston MV. Physiological and pathophysiological roles of excitatory amino acids during central nervous system development. Brain Res Rev 1990;15:41–70.

[51] Lovell MR, Collins MW, Iverson GL, et al. Recovery from mild concussion in high school athletes. J Neurosurg 2003;98:296–301.
[52] Lovell MR, Collins MW, Iverson GL, et al. Grade 1 or "ding" concussion in high school athletes. Am J Sports Med 2004;32(1):47–54.
[53] Farace E, Alves W. Do women fare worse: a meta-analysis of gender differences in traumatic brain injury outcome. J Neurosurg 2000;93:539–45.
[54] Barnes BC, Cooper L, Kirkendall DT, et al. Concussion history in elite male and female soccer players. Am J Sports Med 1998;26(3):433–8.
[55] Roof RL, Duvdevani R, Stein DG. Gender influences outcome of brain injury: progesterone plays a protective role. Brain Res 1993;607:333–6.
[56] Roof RL, Hall ED. Estrogen-related gender differences in survival rate and cortical blood flow after impact acceleration head injury in rats. J Neurotrauma 2000;17:367–88.
[57] Rogers E, Wagner AW. Gender, sex steroids, and neuroprotection following traumatic brain injury. J Head Trauma Rehabil 2006;21(3):279–81.
[58] Stein DG, Hoffman SW. Estrogen and progesterone as neuroprotective agents in the treatment of acute brain injuries. Pediatr Rehabil 2003;6(1):13–22.
[59] Emerson CS, Hadrick JP, Vink R. Estrogen improves biochemical and neurologic outcome following traumatic brain injury in male rats, but not in females. Brain Res 1993;8:95–100.
[60] Iverson G. Predicting slow recovery from sports-related concussion: the new simple-complex distinction. Clin J Sport Med 2007;17:31–7.

ELSEVIER
SAUNDERS

Phys Med Rehabil Clin N Am
19 (2008) 271–285

PHYSICAL MEDICINE
AND REHABILITATION
CLINICS OF
NORTH AMERICA

Shoulder and Elbow Injuries
in the Adolescent Athlete

Brian J. Krabak, MD, MBA[a],*, Eric Alexander, MD[b],
Troy Henning, MD[b]

[a]Rehabilitation, Orthopaedics and Sports Medicine, Team Consultation,
University of Washington Medicine Sports and Spine, 1959 NE Pacific Street,
Box 356490, Seattle, WA 98195, USA
[b]Rehabilitation Medicine, University of Washington, 1959 NE Pacific Street,
Box 356490, Seattle, WA 98195, USA

Shoulder and elbow pain in the adolescent population is different than in the adult population. The difference relates to the immature bone structure of the shoulder and elbow region. although beyond the scope of this article, it is important to understand the maturation of the physis or growth plates. In brief, the physis or epiphyseal plate is where future bone is laid down and is constantly changing during the years of growth. The relative weakness at the physis and decreased resistance to shear and tensile forces compared with the surrounding ligaments, tendons, and muscles predispose this area to potential injury [1]. It is important to take into account maturation of the bone, including the closing of ossification centers, when evaluating the immature athlete. Important ages to remember for closure of the ossifications centers of the shoulder and elbow region include the upper part of the glenoid (16–18 years), the proximal humerus (17–18 years), the lateral epicondyle (14–16 years), and the medial epicondyle (14–16 years).

Specific shoulder and elbow injuries in the adolescent athlete vary from sport to sport. Athletes who play baseball and tennis most commonly experience such pain. Lyman and colleagues [2] noted that 26 to 35 per 100 youth baseball pitchers experienced a shoulder or elbow injury or both during the course of a season. Similarly, 30% of pitchers experienced shoulder pain, and 25% experienced elbow pain after a specific game [3]. In adolescent elite national tennis players (boys aged 16 to 18 years and girls aged 16 years), more than 20% to 45% of all injuries were located in the upper extremity

* Corresponding author.
E-mail address: bkrabak@u.washington.edu (B.J. Krabak).

[4]. Of these athletes, 25% to 30% had previous or current shoulder pain, and 22% to 25% had previous or current elbow pain.

Potential risk factors for subsequent injury depend on the exact sport. In the throwing athlete, risk factors include the number of pitches thrown in a game, the type of pitches, and the number of months pitched in a year [4,5]. These findings have led to recommendations such as limiting the pitch count to less than 80 throws per game, limiting the use of curve balls and sliders, and pitching for less than 8 months in a year to avoid injury [6]. Other studies have started looking at the differences in pitching kinematics and kinetics in adolescent throwers compared with adults to identify bio-mechanic factors that may contribute to overuse and fatigue [7]. Further studies are needed, however. This article reviews several specific injuries to upper extremities in the adolescent athlete.

Glenohumeral instability

In the adolescent population, the shoulder is one of the most unstable joints of the body [8]. Because of the anatomic design of the shoulder joint and immature muscle development, athletes may experience instability caused by dislocation or subluxation. Most commonly, the mechanism of injury is a traumatic event leading to recurrence dislocations. Lawton's [9] review of shoulder instability in athletes aged 16 years and younger reported an initial traumatic event in 86% of athletes. Instability was associated with male sex, adolescence, and a history of trauma. In the skeletally mature adolescent athlete, traumatic dislocations are typically unilateral in nature and treated surgically because of high recurrence rates (80%–90%) [9,10]. Care must be taken when evaluating the skeletally immature shoulder, however, because a traumatic dislocation is more likely to result in a fracture of the proximal humerus. Less commonly, the adolescent athlete may experience atraumatic dislocations in the setting of hypermobile joints and ligamentous laxity. Atraumatic dislocations are typically multidirectional in nature and can be treated with rehabilitation (initially) or surgically [11]. Other athletes, such as baseball pitchers, experience more subtle instability secondary to overuse and weakness of the rotator cuff muscles [5].

Traumatic instability

Anterior dislocations
Anterior dislocations represent more than 90% of traumatic dislocations [8,10]. These injuries are commonly seen in skeletally mature adolescents who participate in contact sports but also may occur when a person hits the ground. The dislocation occurs after a high-energy injury that involves a fall on the outstretched hand while the shoulder is in abduction and external rotation [12]. The athlete may report a "dead arm" caused by a transient loss of sensation or numbness in the involved extremity [12]. The axillary nerve is the most commonly injured structure, and has been involved in

5% to 35% of traumatic anterior shoulder dislocations [10]. The anteriorly dislocating humeral head and joint capsule may tear the labrum from the rim of the glenoid, which leads to a Bankart lesion [13]. Impaction of the posterior humeral head with the anterior glenoid rim leads to a Hill-Sachs lesion that can be seen on plain radiographs. Unfortunately, evidence of a Hill-Sachs lesion carries a worse prognosis for anterior instability secondary to decreased bony support, which is minimal to begin with [13,14].

The diagnosis of anterior shoulder instability frequently is based on the patient's history, physical examination, and radiographic findings. Athletes who experience a traumatic anterior shoulder dislocation often present with an obvious deformity. The humeral head may be visible anteriorly and the acromion may be prominent because of the displaced humeral head. The athlete also holds the arm in an internally rotated position. Results of the anterior apprehension test are considered positive for anterior instability if the patient becomes apprehensive and notes that it feels as though the shoulder is going to slip out of place. Similarly, the anterior drawer test reveals increased displacement of the humeral head anteriorly, which causes apprehension from the athlete.

Diagnostic imaging is necessary to evaluate the integrity of the glenohumeral joint. Radiographs should be performed in multiple planes to properly assess for any dislocation and concurrent fractures. Typical views include the anteroposterior view with the shoulder in internal and external rotation, an axillary or modified axillary view, and the scapular Y view. The modified axillary view—or "West Point" view—is helpful in assessing anterior instability because it gives an excellent view of the glenoid rim to evaluate for a Bankart lesion [13,15]. In the case of an anterior dislocation, radiographs reveal an anteriorly displaced humeral head or Hill-Sachs lesion. If there are no concurrent fractures, then the shoulder may be relocated safely via various techniques. Subsequent MRI may be helpful in evaluating the integrity of labrum or rotator cuff muscles but is more helpful in the evaluation of chronic dislocations.

The initial treatment of an anterior dislocation involves closed reduction with or without anesthesia. Reduction should be accomplished as soon as possible because athletes who have had a dislocation for several hours experience significant pain and muscle spasm that may require an intravenous narcotic and benzodiazepine. Two commonly used techniques for reduction of anterior dislocations are the modified Kocher method and the Stimson method [16]. The modified Kocher method is performed by placing the patient in the supine position with the body stabilized and applying traction on the humerus while the arm is in an adducted, externally rotated, flexed position. If spontaneous reduction is not accomplished with this technique, the arm is then internally rotated and further adducted. In the Stimson technique, the patient lies in the prone position and a weight is placed on the dislocated arm. The humerus should spontaneously return to its normal position in 5 to 15 minutes with the aid of gravity. A detailed postreduction physical examination should be performed and postreduction radiographs should be obtained to confirm reduction and evaluate for any fractures. After reduction, the arm should be immobilized for 2 to 6 weeks in a sling with gradual range-of-motion and strengthening exercises as tolerated [10,17].

Surgical treatment is typically recommended because of the high recurrence rate of instability in young athletes. Several studies have shown decreased rates of recurrent instability and improved outcomes in patients treated with surgical stabilization of acute, traumatic anterior shoulder dislocation when compared with nonoperative treatment in the adolescent population [10,11,18,19]. Lawton [9] retrospectively reviewed the outcome of surgery versus therapy in 70 cases of shoulder instability in athletes aged 16 years and younger. At more than 2-year follow-up, 70% of the surgical group described their shoulders as better and 90% were performing at preinjury levels at sports. Surgically treated patients were less likely to have recurrent stability or report limitations in function. Others have noted an incidence of recurrent dislocation in only 10% to 20% after arthroscopic surgery [18,19]. Jones and Wiesel [20] found primary arthroscopic Bankart repair to be an effective treatment of traumatically induced shoulder instability in pediatric patients. They felt that primary arthroscopic Bankart repair limits multiple recurring shoulder dislocations, which can hinder a patient's quality of life and places them at risk for future negative sequelae. Finally, Jakobsen and Johannsen [21] performed a level I, high-quality, prospective, randomized controlled trial that compared long-term results after surgical and conservative primary treatment of first-time traumatic anterior shoulder dislocation. The results revealed that open repair produces superior results compared with conservative treatment in active patients to reduce the risk of recurrence [21]. Although a discussion of the comparison is beyond the scope of this article, open and arthroscopic surgeries seem to result in similar outcomes [19].

Posterior dislocations

Traumatic posterior dislocation is an uncommon injury that represents less than 5% of all traumatic shoulder dislocations [22]. Posterior dislocation may occur as the result of a fall on the outstretched hand with the shoulder in adduction and internal rotation or direct anterior trauma to the shoulder that forces the humeral head out the back of the glenoid cavity. In football, offensive linemen are particularly vulnerable to this injury because of the forward-flexed and internally rotated shoulder position needed for blocking [23]. On examination, the hallmark of posterior dislocation is loss of external rotation of the shoulder along with prominence of the humeral head on the posterior shoulder [13]. Some athletes may not have any obvious deformity, however, which leads to a missed diagnosis. On examination, the athletes experience apprehension with posterior displacement of the glenohumeral joint. They also complain of posterior shoulder pain and have limited external rotation of the shoulder with forward flexion less than 90°. Radiographs should be obtained in multiple planes, and they typically reveal a posteriorly displaced humeral head.

Recurrent posterior subluxation of the shoulder can be treated successfully with a rotator cuff rehabilitation program, resulting in a variable ability of the patient to return to sports [24]. Surgery is indicated in patients whose function is still markedly impaired after a rehabilitation program. Operative treatment that corrects the underlying pathology is being increasingly offered at an earlier stage to patients whose symptoms are refractory to nonoperative measures [25].

Atraumatic instability

Multidirectional instability

Unlike unilateral instability of the shoulder, multidirectional glenohumeral instability is typically atraumatic in onset. Athletes typically have generalized joint laxity in association with rotator cuff weakness in sports that require overhead arm motions [26,27]. Sports include gymnastics and swimming, in which hypermobile joints may help in competition. The athletes tend to complain of nonspecific shoulder pain and a feeling of shoulder subluxation or dislocation with overhead activities. On physical examination, they have evidence of generalized ligamentous laxity, including hyperextension at the elbows, the ability to approximate the thumbs to the forearms, and hyperextension of the metacarpophalangeal joints [28]. In addition to a positive apprehension sign, physical examination reveals a positive sulcus sign, which indicates inferior instability. Finally, athletes typically experience strength deficits localized to the scapular stabilizers and rotator cuff muscles.

Treatment for multidirectional instability focuses on a customized rehabilitation program. Because most athletes with multidirectional instability have hyperlaxity, stretching of the shoulder joint is typically not necessary. Strengthening exercises focus on the strength deficits noted previously. The initial program includes isometric to isotonic exercises for the scapular stabilizers (the serratus anterior, pectoralis, and latissimus dorsi muscles) and rotator cuff muscles [29,30]. These exercises then progress to more integrative and functional activities specific to the athlete's sport. Posterior and multidirectional instability usually responds to conservative treatment with physical therapy for rehabilitation, unless a specific anatomic lesion is noted [26,27]. Most of the patients who respond favorably to conservative treatment show a positive response within 3 months of beginning a rehabilitation program [31]. Patients who have unilateral involvement, impairment of daily activities, and high grades of laxity have a greater likelihood of requiring surgery than their counterparts [31]. Any athlete with multidirectional instability who continues to experience dislocation or subluxation after conservative treatment should be referred for surgery for a possible inferior capsular shift.

Adolescent athlete's shoulder and proximal humeral epiphysiolysis

Proximal humeral epiphysiolysis, also known as Little League shoulder and more recently referred to as adolescent athletes shoulder by Johnson and Houchin [32], is a repetitive strain injury to the proximal humeral epiphysis. It generally occurs in adolescents between the ages of 11 and 15. Overtraining and improper biomechanics seen in over-head sports lead to repetitive stress and rotational torques that eventually compromise the physis. Baseball primarily has been the focus of studies looking at this phenomenon; however, it also can be seen in sports such as volleyball, swimming, and badminton [33]. Typically, patients note pain at the superior lateral aspect of the shoulder with dynamic/resisted over-head activities that simulate competition-level intensities. On examination, palpation along the area of the proximal humeral epiphysis is tender. Active range of motion is usually full and pain free. Resisted strength testing in a functional/over-head position or while inducing torque within the humerus generally reproduces the pain.

Radiographic visualization of the physis injury is best demonstrated on anteroposterior comparison views of the proximal humerus with the arm internally and externally rotated [34]. External rotation views show widening of the physis at the lateral aspect (Fig. 1). Internal rotational views demonstrate two horizontal radiolucent lines [34]. Lateral fragmentation, calcification, sclerosis, and cyst changes also can be seen, with the widening physis typifying its chronic nature [34]. The exact mechanism of physis injury has yet to be determined; however, it is thought to resemble a Salter Harris type 1 fracture with separation of the metaphysic from the epiphysis. Some investigators have postulated that chronic stress injury leads to an alteration in the endochondral ossification center and delay in apoptosis.

Yamamoto and colleagues [35] recently analyzed humeral retroversion in adolescent baseball players and found a significantly increased amount of

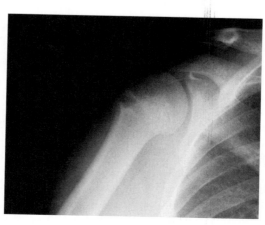

Fig. 1. Radiograph of an adolescent shoulder showing widening of the physis, laterally.

retroversion in the dominant arm compared with the nondominant arm. It is generally thought that with normal development the amount of retroversion should decrease with age. Yamamoto and colleagues contributed their findings to a delay in derotation of the humerus caused by repetitive throwing activities. They also found that players who began pitching before age 11 had a greater degree of retroversion (although not statistically significant) than players who started after age 11. These findings, along with radiographic evidence of degenerative changes, point more toward a gradual microtrauma mechanism than an acute fracture. As a result, it is not uncommon for radiographic evidence of closure to take 9 to 12 months, which distinguishes it from a typical (acute) Salter Harris fracture [34].

Treatment is generally based on professional experience rather than rigorous studies. Eliminating painful activities while allowing the athlete to use other positions or cross-train until pain free is typical. Because radiographic evidence of physis closure can take several months, it is typically not used as a marker of when to return to offending activities. Once patients can perform over-head activities in a pain-free manner, they are gradually allowed to return to play. Physical therapy is usually not needed and, in some case reports, leads to worsening of pain [34]. Overall, the best treatment is to prevent injury in the first place. In a recent review by Caine and colleagues [33], several essential goals were outlined clearly, including proper education of the athlete, parents, coaches, and other training persons and appropriate training practices, skill development, and periodization.

Rotator cuff injuries

In adolescent athletes, injury to the rotator cuff muscles is rare, occurring in less than 1% of athletes younger than 20 years of age [36]. They are usually the result of an acute traumatic event, secondary impingement because of poor muscular/proprioceptive control, or internal impingement caused by tightness of the posterior capsule/shoulder soft tissue structures. Traumatic events typically involve falling onto an outstretched arm or forcibly impacting an immoveable object (ie, hitting the boards in hockey).

Unlike adults, secondary impingement occurs because of nonoutlet diseases leading to external or internal impingement. Nonoutlet diseases include bursal thickening, contracture of the posterior capsule, and instability of the glenohumeral joint [37–39]. It is believed that subtle instability of the glenohumeral joint and poor muscle control of the rotator cuff muscles cause a deficiency in the compressive forces needed to stabilize the glenohumeral during over-head movements. This instability allows for repeated contact of the supraspinatus and/or subscapularis against the acrominon or coracoacromial arch, respectively. In the case of internal impingement, it is thought to occur as a result of excessive tightness of the posterior shoulder capsule or overlying musculature. Inappropriate biomechanics lead to the inappropriate contact of the posterior region of the supraspinatus and superior aspect of the infraspinatus tendon with the posterior glenoid rim, which results in a partial-thickness tearing of the undersurface (articular side) of these tendons and fraying of the posterior superior glenoid labrum. Athletes with this form of impingement describe posterior shoulder pain along with decreased throwing/hitting endurance, accuracy, and velocity.

Evaluation of adolescent shoulder injuries should include a detailed history and examination of the shoulder complex. In the throwing athlete, care should be taken to review the pitch count, types of pitches, and amount of pitching throughout the year because these factors have been shown to increase the risk of shoulder injury [38,39]. Physical examination should include inspection, palpation, range-of-motion testing, neurologic assessment, and stress testing of the rotator cuff muscle group, biceps, labrum, and capsule. It is also important to review the biomechanical motions of the shoulder relevant to the specific sport. Itoi and colleagues [40] found that in most patients with rotator cuff tears, location of pain is a poor predictor of which rotator cuff muscle was injured. They found manual muscle testing of the supraspinatus, infraspinatus, and subscapularis to be a more reliable indicator. Motor examination scores of less than 5/5, 4+/5, and 3/5, respectively, correlated well with arthroscopic findings. Similar to adults, imaging of the shoulder complex with MRI or even ultrasound typically identifies the type of tear.

Treatment of rotator cuff pathology depends on the severity of the tear. In general, adolescent athletes can be treated conservatively with cessation of the aggravating injury and a focused therapy program. In pitchers, time should be taken to review the pitch count, types of pitches, and amount of pitching throughout the year. Therapy should focus on strengthening the scapular stabilizers and rotator cuff muscles. The motions should be integrated into a functional analysis of the pitching biomechanics. After any abnormal motions are corrected, athletes may slowly increase their velocity and return to sport as tolerated.

Osteochondritis dissecans of the elbow (Little League elbow)

Osteochondritis dissecans of the capitellum is the leading cause of permanent elbow disability in adolescent athletes [41]. There are two main types of osteochondritis dissecans: the adult form, which occurs after the physis closes, and the juvenile form, which occurs in patients with an open epiphyseal plate. With immature bone structure and relatively weak physes, the adolescent elbow often presents an injury pattern different from that in the elbow of the mature athlete. Humeral capitellum osteochondritis dissecans or Little League elbow is believed to affect 4 of every 1000 boys [42]. It usually occurs in the dominant arm, and in up to 20% of cases, it occurs bilaterally [41]. In this article we concentrate on the juvenile form of osteochondritis dissecans.

Osteochondritis dissecans is characterized by a focal area of subchondral bone that undergoes necrosis. The disease causes a section of joint surface cartilage and the bone beneath it to loosen and from the main or "parent" bone structure [43]. It may result directly from trauma or secondarily from loss of blood supply to an area of subchondral bone, resulting in avascular necrosis. As the necrotic bone is resorbed, the overlying cartilage loses its support. Without its cartilage cover, the bony fragment may become dislodged into the joint. These fragments of cartilage or bone become loose within a joint, leading to pain and inflammation. The fragments are sometimes referred to as "joint mice" because of a squeaking sound sometimes resulting from the joint [43]. The actual cause of osteochondritis dissecans is commonly believed to be multifactorial, with repetitive microtrauma to the immature capitellum during throwing playing an instigating role [44]. After tendinopathies and posterior impingement, osteochondritis dissecans is the most common injury of the elbow in athletes [45].

Accurate diagnosis depends on understanding the anatomy and sports biomechanics of an athlete's elbow, because athletes often complain of pain during sporting activity but are asymptomatic during daily life [46–48]. Most individuals with capitellar osteochondritis dissecans are young male Little League baseball pitchers or female gymnasts who present with pain, tenderness, and swelling over the lateral aspect of the elbow. Players continue to play baseball because their elbow pain is not severe enough to warrant medical attention. Specifically for throwing athletes, any changes in accuracy, velocity, stamina, and strength are important in the history. Patients usually report pain at the extremes of motion range. It also commonly occurs in persons who participate in racquet sports and weightlifting. Typically, there is no history of trauma. An insidious onset of dull, activity-related, and poorly localized pain may precede other more severe symptoms, such as locking, decreased motion, and flexion contracture of more than 15° [42]. Subtle restriction in range of motion may be the most important clinical sign. On examination, effusions, crepitus, and joint line tenderness may be present [44]. Periarticular edema often is present with slight warmth to the touch.

Clinical findings may be subtle, so clinicians should have a low threshold of suspicion for obtaining radiographs. Early diagnosis and appropriate management may prevent long-term sequelae. On conventional radiographs, osteochondral lesions may appear normal [49]. When detectable, osteochondral lesions appear as lucencies in the articular epiphysis (Fig. 2). In longstanding disease, flattening of the capitellum and nondisplaced fragmentation of the subchondral bone or even focal defects of the capitellum with loose bodies can be seen on an anteroposterior radiograph of the elbow. MRI, preferably with arthrography, is the first choice for evaluating osteochondritis dissecans. Sensitivities up to 95% have been reported [49]. MRI can detect the presence of osteochondritis dissecans in the early stages of the disease process when radiographs are normal or show only subtle changes in the appearance of the capitellum [50]. MRI also may provide useful information about the size, location, and stability of the osteochondritis dissecans lesion (Fig. 3). These factors are all important when determining the best treatment option in patients with osteochondritis dissecans of the capitellum [51]. Unstable

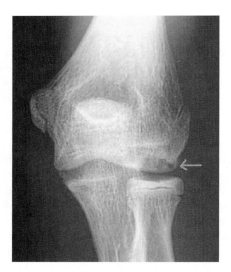

Fig. 2. Radiograph of an adolescent elbow showing an osteochondral defect (*arrow*).

osteochondritis dissecans lesions are surrounded by a rim of high signal intensity or a fluid-filled cyst on T2-weighted images. Stable osteochondritis dissecans lesions show no surrounding signal abnormality on T2-weighted images. Nuclear medicine, scintigraphic findings are nonspecific, demonstrating

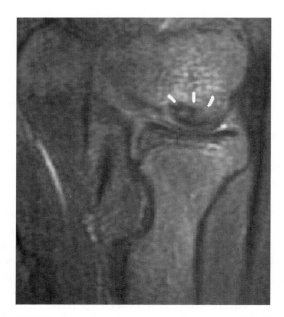

Fig. 3. MRI T2 of the elbow showing an osteochondral defect (*marks*).

a mild-to-marked increase in focal uptake in the involved bone, depending on the age of the osteochondritis dissecans. Recently, sonography, which is a safe, inexpensive, and portable type of diagnostic imaging, has been used to assess elbow injuries [52]. Sonography can be performed on the field where athletes are training or playing, so it might be possible to detect and treat elbow injuries before they become advanced [53]. Osteochondritis dissecans can be detected by sonography even in its asymptomatic stage [53].

Treatment of capitellar osteochondritis dissecans is somewhat controversial but begins with staging of the lesion. MRI is the most accurate method for staging lesions, short of arthroscopy, which bases the classification on the appearance of the overlying articular cartilage. MRI classification of osteochondritis dissecans is (I) marrow edema (stable), (II) breach of articular cartilage, with low-signal rim surrounding fragment indicating fibrous attachment (stable), (III) pockets of fluid around undetached and undisplaced osteochondral fragment (unstable), and (IV) displaced osteochondral fragment (unstable) [54]. Once classified, available treatment options are determined. An osteochondritis dissecans lesion of the capitellum can be classified as stable or unstable [54]. A stable lesion is one that can heal completely with elbow rest, and an unstable lesion is one for which surgery provides significantly better results.

Conservative treatment (low-intensity physical rehabilitation) is recommended for stable (stages I and II) lesions. If symptoms worsen or fail to improve or crepitus develops (suggesting detachment), then arthroscopy is recommended to evaluate stability of the lesion. Depending on findings at arthroscopy, a loose body may be removed, a fragment may be excised, cartilage may be debrided, or a lesion may be drilled to promote revascularization.

Nonoperative methods of treatment for osteochondritis dissecans of the capitellum include activity modification and periods of immobilization (6- to 8-week break from competitive sports) followed by therapy and range-of-motion exercises [55]. Once symptoms have decreased, active range of motion is begun and the elbow is protected until radiographic confirmation of revascularization or healing [55]. If symptoms persist over 8 to 12 weeks and the lesion demarcates on MRI, arthroscopic or open subchondral drilling is indicated [5]. Prognosis worsens with age and physis closure. The goal of management of osteochondritis dissecans is to promote resolution of the lesion before physis closure [42]. Some studies have shown that early capitellar lesions can resolve with activity modification and rest if the defect is diagnosed early in its development [56]. Other studies show fair to poor results in conservatively treated osteochondritis dissecans of the elbow [57]. The role of physiotherapy and nonsteroidal anti-inflammatory drugs remains unclear.

Surgical treatment may be indicated if there are persistent symptoms, a loose body, or approaching skeletal maturity or if MRI reveals a fracture through the articular cartilage [58]. Possible surgical procedures are open débridement, subchondral drilling, bone grafting, refixation, chondral transplantation, and osteotomy [52,59,60]. Another option is arthroscopic débridement, which may provide less operative morbidity with earlier return to activity than arthrotomy [55]. After surgery, range-of-motion exercises should be initiated early. Patients should be followed at 3-month intervals with a clinical history and physical examination until symptoms resolve.

Prevention

The key in the treatment of osteochondritis dissecans is prevention, and this responsibility is widespread. Emphasis must be placed on preseason conditioning, proper throwing mechanics, and proper warm-up exercises. There are three main contributors to a young pitcher's ability to stay healthy: pitching mechanics, pitching type, and pitching volume [61]. Proper throwing and pitching mechanics must be emphasized at an early age to help reduce this risk. In a recent prospective study of 298 youth baseball players, arm fatigue and more than 600 pitches thrown per season were found to be risk factors for elbow pain [2]. Little League, Inc. guidelines relate to the number of innings pitched per week: less than six innings/week for the 9- to 12-year-old group and less than nine innings/week for the 13- to 15-year-old group. Some authors have emphasized the number of actual pitches thrown in practice and in games: less than 75 pitches/game, less than 600 pitches/season [2]. No suggestions found in the literature are evidence based. The issue is likely multifactorial; not only is the cumulative amount of pitches thrown important but also the type of pitches thrown, the position played, and perhaps most importantly, the technique and subsequent position of the elbow at ball release [2].

Summary

Adolescent athletes may experience various unique injuries to the shoulder and elbow. It is important for sports medicine physicians to appreciate the various stresses and impact of each sport on possible injury. Expedient diagnosis allows more efficient treatment, quicker recovery, and prevention of any future injuries during the athlete's career.

References

[1] Wojtys EM. Sports injuries in the immature athlete. Orthop Clin North Am 1987;18(4): 689–708.

[2] Lyman S, Fleisig GS, Waterbor JW, et al. Longitudinal study of elbow and shoulder pain in youth baseball pitchers. Med Sci Sports Exerc 2001;33:1803–10.

[3] Lyman S, Fleisig GS, Andrews JR, et al. Effect of pitch type, pitch count, and pitching mechanics on risk of elbow and shoulder pain in youth baseball pitchers. Am J Sports Med 2002;30:463–8.

[4] Safran MR, Hutchinson MR, Moss R, et al. A comparison of injuries in elite boys and girls tennis players. Transactions of the 9th Annual Meeting of the Society of Tennis Medicine and Science, Indian Wells, CA; 1999.

[5] Kocher MS, Walters PM, Micheli LJ. Upper extremity injuries in the paediatric athlete [review]. Sports Med 2000;30(2):117–35.

[6] Olsen SJ 2nd, Fleisig GS, Dun S, et al. Risk factors for shoulder and elbow injuries in adolescent baseball pitchers. Am J Sports Med 2006;34(6):905–12.

[7] Nissen CW, Westwell M, Ounpus S, et al. Adolescent baseball pitching technique: a detailed three-dimensional biomechanical analysis. Med Sci Sports Exerc 2007;39(8):1347–57.

[8] Mahaffey BL, Smith PA. Shoulder instability in young athletes. Am Fam Physician 1999;59: 2773–82.

[9] Lawton RL, Choudhury S, Mansat P, et al. Pediatric shoulder instability: presentation, findings, treatment, and outcomes. J Pediatr Orthop 2002;22:52–61.

[10] Good CR, MacGillivray JD. Traumatic shoulder dislocation in the adolescent athlete: advances in surgical treatment. Curr Opin Pediatr 2005;17:25–9.

[11] Stein DA, Jazrawi L, Bartolozzi AR. Arthroscopic stabilization of anterior shoulder instability: a review of the literature. Arthroscopy 2002;18(8):912–24.

[12] Bahr R, Craig EV, Engebretsen L. The clinical presentation of shoulder instability including on field management. Clin Sports Med 1995;14:761–76.

[13] Allen AA, Warner JJ. Shoulder instability in the athlete. Orthop Clin North Am 1995;26: 487–504.

[14] Liu SH, Henry MH. Anterior shoulder instability: current review. Clin Orthop 1996;323: 327–37.

[15] Jahnke AH Jr, Petersen SA, Neumann C, et al. A prospective comparison of computerized arthrotomography and magnetic resonance imaging of the glenohumeral joint. Am J Sports Med 1992;20:695–700.

[16] McKeag DB, McCoy RL. Common injuries in the child or adolescent athlete. Prim Care 1995;22(1):114–44.

[17] Patterson PD, Waters PM. Shoulder injuries in the child athlete. Clin Sports Med 2000;19(4): 681–92.

[18] Arciero RA, St. Pierre P. Acute shoulder dislocation: indications and techniques for operative management. Clin Sports Med 1995;14:937–53.

[19] Guanche CA, Quick DC, Sodergren KM, et al. Arthroscopic versus open reconstruction of the shoulder in patients with isolated Bankart lesions. Am J Sports Med 1996;24:144–8.

[20] Jones KJ, Wiesel B. Functional outcomes of early arthroscopic Bankart repair in adolescents aged 11 to 18 years. J Pediatr Orthop 2007;27(2):209–13.

[21] Jakobsen BW, Johannsen HV. Primary repair versus conservative treatment of first-time traumatic anterior dislocation of the shoulder: a randomized study with 10-year follow-up. Arthroscopy 2007;23(2):118–23.

[22] Kawam M, Sinclair J, Letts M. Recurrent posterior shoulder dislocation in children: the results of surgical management. J Pediatr Orthop 1997;17:533–8.

[23] Tibone JE, Bradley JP. The treatment of posterior subluxation in athletes. Clin Orthop 1993; 291:124–37.

[24] Hurley JA, Anderson TE. Posterior shoulder instability: surgical versus conservative results with evaluation of glenoid version. Am J Sports Med 1992;20:396–400.

[25] Papendick LW, Savoie FH. Anatomy-specific repair techniques for posterior shoulder instability. J South Orthop Assoc 1995;4:169–76.

[26] Friedman RJ, Blocker ER, Morrow DL. Glenohumeral instability. J South Orthop Assoc 1995;4:182–99.

[27] Yamaguchi K, Flatow EL. Management of multidirectional instability. Clin Sports Med 1995;14:885–902.

[28] Cordasco FA. Understanding multidirectional instability of the shoulder. J Athl Train 2000; 35(3):278–85.

[29] Burkhead WZ, Rockwood CA. Treatment of instability of the shoulder with an exercise program. J Bone Joint Surg Am 1992;74:890–6.

[30] Kibler WB, Rubin RD. Fundamental principles of shoulder rehabilitation: conservative to postoperative management. Arthroscopy 2002;18:29–39.

[31] Misamore GW, Sallay PI. A longitudinal study of patients with multidirectional instability of the shoulder with seven- to ten-year follow-up. J Shoulder Elbow Surg 2005;14(5):466–70.

[32] Johnson J, Houchin G. Adolescent athlete's shoulder: a case series. Clin J Sport Med 2006; 16:84–6.

[33] Caine D, DiFiori J, Maffulli N. Physeal injuries in children's and youth sports: reasons for concern? Br J Sports Med 2006;40:749–60.

[34] Carson W, Gasser S. Little Leaguer's shoulder: case report. Am J Sports Med 1998;26: 575–80.

[35] Yamamoto N, Itoi E, Minagawa H, et al. Why is the humeral retroversion of throwing athletes greater in dominant shoulders than in nondominant shoulders? J Shoulder Elbow Surg 2006;15(5):571–5.

[36] Tarkin IS. Rotator cuff tears in adolescent athletes. Am J Sports Med 2005;33:596–601.

[37] Ong BC, Sekiya JK, Rodosky MW. Shoulder injuries in the athlete. Curr Opin Rheumatol 2002;14:150–9.

[38] Lyman S, Fleisig GS, Andrews JR, et al. Effect of pitch type, pitch count, and pitching mechanics on risk of elbow and shoulder pain in youth baseball pitchers. Am J Sports Med 2002;33(4):463–8.

[39] Olsen SJ, Fleisig GS, Dun S, et al. Risk factors for shoulder and elbow injuries in adolescent baseball pitchers. Am J Sports Med 2006;34(6):905–12.

[40] Itoi E, Minagawa H, Yamamoto N, et al. Are pain location and physical examinations useful in locating a tear site of the rotator cuff? Am J Sports Med 2006;34:256–64.

[41] Fleisig GS, Barrentine SW, Andrews JR, et al. Biomechanics of overhand throwing with implications for injuries. Sports Med 1996;21(6):421–37.

[42] Klingele KE, Kocher MS. Little League elbow: valgus overload injury in the paediatric athlete. Sports Med 2002;32:1005–15.

[43] Clanton TO, DeLee JC. Osteochondritis dissecans: history, pathophysiology and current treatment concepts. Clin Orthop Relat Res 1982;167:50–64.

[44] Williamson LR, Albright JP. Bilateral osteochondritis dissecans of the elbow in a female pitcher. J Fam Pract 1996;43:489–93.

[45] Williams RJ 3rd, Urquhart ER, Altchek DW. Medial collateral ligament tears in the throwing athlete. Instr Course Lect 2004;53:579–86.

[46] Eygendaal D, Olsen BS, Jensen SL, et al. Kinematics of partial and total ruptures of the medial collateral ligament of the elbow. J Shoulder Elbow Surg 1999;8:612–6.

[47] Eygendaal D, Heijboer MP, Obermann WR, et al. Medial instability of the elbow: findings on valgus load radiography and MRI in 16 athletes. Acta Orthop Scand 2000;71:480–3.

[48] Eygendaal D. Ligamentous reconstruction around the elbow using triceps tendon. Acta Orthop Scand 2004;75:516–23.

[49] Potter HG. Imaging of posttraumatic and soft tissue dysfunction of the elbow. Clin Orthop Relat Res 2000;370:9–18.

[50] Cugat R, Garcia M, Cusco X, et al. Osteochondritis dissecans: a historical review and its treatment with cannulated screws. Arthroscopy 1993;9:675–84.

[51] Kiyoshige Y, Takagi M, Yuasa K, et al. Closed-wedge osteotomy for osteochondritis dissecans of the capitellum: a 7- to 12-year follow-up. Am J Sports Med 2000;28:534–7.

[52] Sasaki J, Takahara M, Ogino T, et al. Ultrasonographic assessment of the ulnar collateral ligament and medial elbow laxity in college baseball players. J Bone Joint Surg Am 2002; 84:525–31.

[53] Harada M, Takahara M, Sasaki J, et al. Using sonography for the early detection of elbow injuries among young baseball players. Am J Roentgenol 2006;187:1436–41.

[54] Takahara M. Classification, treatment, and outcome of osteochondritis dissecans of the humeral capitellum. J Bone Joint Surg Am 2007;89:1205–14.

[55] Bradley JP, Petrie RS. Osteochondritis dissecans of the humeral capitellum: diagnosis and treatment. Clin Sports Med 2001;20:565–90.

[56] Yadao MA, Field LD, Savoie FH 3rd. Osteochondritis dissecans of the elbow. Instr Course Lect 2004;53:599–606.

[57] Takahara M, Ogino T, Fukushima S, et al. Nonoperative treatment of osteochondritis dissecans of the humeral capitellum. Am J Sports Med 1999;27:728–32.

[58] Pill SG, Ganley TJ, Flynn JM, et al. Osteochondritis dissecans of the capitellum: arthroscopic-assisted treatment of large, full-thickness defects in young patients. Arthroscopy 2003;19(2): 222–5.

[59] McManama GB Jr, Micheli LJ, Berry MV, et al. The surgical treatment of osteochondritis of the capitellum. Am J Sports Med 1985;13:11–21.

[60] Shimada K, Yoshida T, Nakata K, et al. Reconstruction with an osteochondral autograft for advanced osteochondritis dissecans of the elbow. Clin Orthop Relat Res 2005;435:140–7.

[61] Andrews JR, Fleisig GS. Preventing throwing injuries. J Orthop Sports Phys Ther 1998; 27(3):187–8.

ELSEVIER
SAUNDERS

Phys Med Rehabil Clin N Am
19 (2008) 287–304

PHYSICAL MEDICINE
AND REHABILITATION
CLINICS OF
NORTH AMERICA

Low Back Pain in the Adolescent Athlete

Christopher J. Standaert, MD

*Departments of Rehabilitation Medicine, Orthopaedic and Sports Medicine,
and Neurological Surgery, University of Washington, 325 9th Avenue,
Box 359721, Seattle, WA 98104, USA*

Treating adolescent athletes who have low back pain (LBP) can be a challenging clinical undertaking. From a medical standpoint, adolescents cannot be thought of as merely young adults. The demographics of spinal injury in adolescents are different from those in adults, and some clinical conditions are essentially unique to the adolescent population. The ongoing growth of adolescents introduces variables into care that are not present in the management of adults. Distinct physiologic and cultural issues also affect the diagnosis and management of spinal disorders in adolescents. To treat these athletes appropriately, clinicians must have a working knowledge of spine development, injury patterns and frequencies, and the conditions that are of particular concern in these athletes while being able to manage these conditions over time. Clinicians also must be aware of the psychosocial issues affecting young athletes and be able to work with parents, coaches, and others involved in the ongoing training, support, and performance of the athlete.

The growing spine

The spine in children and adolescents has some distinct structural differences that affect the nature of injury. The nucleus pulposus of a child's spine is relatively more hydrophilic than of an adult, resulting in more effective force absorption and a more central distribution of force transfer to the adjacent vertebrae. The composition of the nucleus pulposus begins to change as early as age 7 or 8 years, and the force distribution of the disc moves more peripherally [1]. The vertebrae each have three primary ossification centers: one in the vertebral body and two in the vertebral arch. The latter typically fuse by 2 to 6 years, and failure of fusion results in a spina bifida occulta [2,3]. Growth of the vertebral body occurs by way of the physes associated with the vertebral end plate. The vertebral end plate is composed

E-mail address: cjs1@u.washington.edu

of hyaline cartilage adjacent to the nucleus pulposus and physeal cartilage adjacent to the vertebral body. The physeal cartilage consists of a ring apophysis and an end plate physis. The ring apophysis surrounds the periphery of the vertebral body and accounts for growth of vertebral body breadth. It begins to ossify at 7 or 8 years old. The end plate physis accounts for the vertical growth of the vertebral body. These physes begin to fuse with the vertebral body at about age 14 to 15 years, with final closure occurring around age 21 to 25 years [1,2]. Biomechanical studies have indicated that the bony strength of the vertebrae, particularly the neural arch, can increase into the fourth or fifth decade of life [4].

There are several aspects of this developmental pattern that are important in understanding injury to the young spine. The more central distribution of force by way of the nucleus pulposus combined with a relatively weak vertebral end plate may account for the relatively high frequency of end plate herniations of disc material (also termed Schmorl's nodes) that occur in children and adolescents compared with adults. The physes themselves may be vulnerable during development, leaving adolescents at risk for apophyseal ring fractures. The relative strength of the intervertebral disc compared with that of the adjacent bone may also account for the relative reduction in rates of discogenic injuries seen in adolescents compared with adults [1–3]. The incomplete bony maturation present in the neural arch also likely contributes to the occurrence of pars fractures in adolescents.

Demographics

LBP is a common occurrence in adolescents, in general, but athletes participating in a number of sports may be at a more substantial risk of pain and structural injury than age-related peers. In general-population studies, the lifetime prevalence of LBP by the midteenage years is 50% or more, with point or 1-year prevalence rates of 17% to 50% [5–10]. The prevalence of LBP increases with age throughout childhood, and a number of studies have reported higher rates of LBP in girls than in boys, although this is not a uniform finding [5–8,10]. The connection between physical activity and LBP is somewhat unclear because studies tend to differ in their findings in this regard [7,10–13]. A study that used an accelerometer to objectively assess activity levels in children and adolescents, however, found no association between LBP and physical activity [13]. A number of studies have identified an association between depression or other emotional problems and LBP in adolescents [14]. A large-scale twin study also identified LBP in adolescence as a significant risk factor for LBP as an adult [15].

The findings in studies of adolescent athletes vary some by sport. Kujala and colleagues [16] noted significantly higher rates of LBP in female gymnasts and figure skaters and in male hockey and soccer players compared with non-athletes (45% versus 18% over 3 years). Sward and colleagues [17] noted that 79% of the male gymnasts they studied had a history of LBP compared with

38% of control subjects. In another study, Sward and colleagues [18] assessed wrestlers, gymnasts, and soccer and tennis players and found that 65% of these athletes had a history of LBP, with male gymnasts having the highest frequency (85%). LBP has also been reported to be a significant problem in golfers, rowers, and rugby players, among others [19–21].

Numerous investigators have also documented high rates of structural abnormalities on imaging studies of young athletes in some sports. In their study on male gymnasts, Sward and colleagues [17] found thoracolumbar disc degeneration on MRI in 75% of the gymnasts compared with 31% of control subjects, Schmorl's nodes in 71% of the gymnasts compared with 44% of the control subjects, and injuries to the ring apophysis in 17% of the gymnasts compared with none of the control subjects. Similarly, Goldstein and colleagues [22] found much higher rates of various structural abnormalities on MRI studies of elite gymnasts compared with elite swimmers. Bennett and colleagues [23] studied elite female gymnasts with MRI and found apophyseal injuries in almost half and disc degeneration in over 60%. Iwamoto and colleagues [21,24] noted structural abnormalities on plain radiographs in over 60% of the high school and collegiate football players they evaluated in one study and in 74% of the rugby players assessed in another study. A number of studies (discussed later) have also shown much higher rates of spondylolysis in high-level adolescent athletes compared with studies in the general population [25–28]. Despite high levels of structural abnormalities on plain films and high rates of reported LBP for young athletes competing in a number of sports, longer-term follow-up studies on many of these athletes do not show any significant increased risk for ongoing LBP into adulthood compared with the general population [29–31].

A general approach to the adolescent athlete who has low back pain

Any young athlete presenting with LBP who is unable to participate in his or her chosen sport because of pain needs to be thoroughly assessed for the presence of significant underlying pathology. Not only are these individuals at risk for a number of structural injuries given their age and activity levels but they are also at risk for a number of "nonmechanical" causes of LBP associated with their age, including disc space infections, neoplasms, inflammatory conditions, and developmental disorders of the spine [32–35]. The development of a rational diagnostic strategy is contingent on understanding the pertinent risks for a given individual; however, vigilance and a certain degree of compulsion are necessary to keep working through potential causes of pain to exclude the more concerning options, particularly when common structural issues are not identified or when athletes are not responding as expected to what seems to be appropriate treatment.

A comprehensive history is the initial step in the evaluation of all young athletes who have LBP. A number of potential risk factors for spinal injury or LBP in athletes have been identified, although some remain controversial.

These risk factors include prior low back or lower-extremity injuries, incomplete rehabilitation of prior injuries, decreased endurance, lower-extremity muscle imbalance, high number of hours of participation per week, and the occurrence of stressful life events. Additional proximate causal factors associated with sports-related injury may include the individual mechanics and skill level associated with sports performance, training patterns, and equipment or facility problems [33,36]. The mode of onset, severity, and progression over time of the individual's symptoms provide useful insight into potential causes. Symptoms that remain relatively mild for an extended period of time before presentation may be suggestive of less significant structural injuries or more indolent underlying processes, whereas more severe, acute, or progressive symptoms may suggest a more substantial structural injury or a rapidly progressive process such as infection. The nature of an athlete's specific sport may also predispose that individual to particular problems, and the timing of injury or pain in relation to the competitive season or training cycle may be relevant for diagnosis and treatment.

Distinctions should also be made regarding additional characteristics of the symptoms. Axial LBP without lower-extremity symptoms should be viewed differently from a presentation that includes leg pain or neurologic dysfunction. The latter symptoms suggest the presence of nerve root or spinal cord involvement, which would make a diagnosis like spondylolysis without spondylolisthesis or an apophyseal injury seem less likely. Bilateral leg pain should suggest bilateral foraminal involvement (such as might be seen with a significant spondylolisthesi), central canal stenosis (such as might be seen with a disc herniation in the setting of a congenitally small spinal canal), or a spinal cord process. Lower-extremity symptoms may also arise from a number of nonspinal sources that should be considered, including diagnoses such as stress fractures, compartment syndrome, or musculotendinous injuries. Pain at night is often thought to be suggestive of an infectious or neoplastic process [35]. The location of the back pain can significantly affect the differential diagnosis. Thoracic or thoracolumbar pain may be associated with discogenic processes or Scheuermann's kyphosis but uncommonly associated with spondylolysis. Low lumbar pain may have many potential causes, including disc or bony sources, whereas sacral pain may be more associated with conditions such as sacroiliitis or a sacral stress fracture, although disc, bone, and nerve root processes in the lower lumbar spine may also result in pain in the sacral region. The presence or absence of associated symptoms can also be helpful in refining the differential diagnosis. Fever, lethargy, weight loss, rashes, headaches, and similar symptoms raise concern for significant systemic processes, including infection and malignancy [34,35]. Morning stiffness or additional joint symptoms may suggest a diffuse inflammatory process.

A thorough history is followed by a comprehensive physical examination structured to identify significant pathology, to work through the differential diagnosis, and to aid in the development of further diagnostic and treatment plans. The physical examination should always include an examination of lumbopelvic motion, palpation of the spine and related structures, and a neurologic examination. It is important to assess a number of other factors in injured athletes, including lower-extremity alignment and function, gait and balance, specific provocative maneuvers, and components of the relevant "kinetic chain" of motion for that athlete. Clearly, other components of a comprehensive physical examination need to be included as medically appropriate. Consideration needs to be given to the potential for significant structural injury, including fracture, and the examination should always be modified appropriately for a given patient to elicit essential information while avoiding further harm.

Spinal imaging is often crucial to establishing a specific diagnosis. Clinicians must be familiar with the strengths and limitations of the different imaging modalities that are available and be comfortable with directly assessing the images. Given the relative sensitivities and specificities of the various diagnostic options, appropriate decisions need to be made regarding which studies are to be obtained, and the findings need to be interpreted in light of the history and physical examination before arriving at a diagnostic conclusion. Imaging strategies (discussed later) may be different for various clinical concerns.

Treatment of adolescent athletes involves a number of specific considerations. The state and demands of physiologic development of the athlete need to be taken into consideration when planning physical training. The psychosocial environment of an injured athlete may also pose challenges for treatment, and the psychologic impact of injury can be difficult for athletes and their families. The use of medications may be problematic. There are limited to no data on the effects on children and adolescents of a number of medications commonly used to manage pain in adults. Care needs to be taken regarding weight and age in prescribing medications to young athletes, and clinicians need to be aware of any potential conflicts with substance use policies that may apply to an athlete's given sport or level of competition. It is unfortunate that there are high rates of use of ergogenic aids and performance-enhancing supplements among adolescent athletes, which introduce the potential for medication interactions, among other problems [37]. The use of these supplements, legal or illegal, may not necessarily be reported to clinicians routinely, and the likelihood of this seems even lower when specific questions regarding their use are not asked.

Specific conditions

There are a number of specific clinical entities that are particularly important to understand in managing young athletes who have LBP. These conditions include spondylolysis, spondylolisthesis, discogenic injuries, and Scheuermann's kyphosis.

Spondylolysis and spondylolisthesis

Spondylolysis should be considered a diagnostic possibility in almost every adolescent athlete who has significant LBP. In a study by Micheli and Wood [38], spondylolysis was the most frequent diagnosis made in adolescent athletes presenting to a sports medicine clinic with LBP. The term *spondylolysis* refers to a defect in the pars interarticularis of the vertebral arch. *Spondylolisthesis* is a separate but related term referring to the anterior displacement of a vertebral body on the one subjacent to it (Fig. 1). Spondylolysis and spondylolisthesis are most frequently viewed under the categorization proposed by Wiltse and colleagues [39], in which the term *isthmic spondylolysis* is used to identify patients who have sustained a lesion in the pars. It is generally believed that the pars lesion in isthmic spondylolysis represents a fatigue fracture of the bone, and most pars lesions identified (85%–95%) occur at L5 [25,26,28,40]. In a study of 4243 young athletes who had LBP, Rossi and Dragoni [27] found that about one half of those who had spondylolysis also had concurrent spondylolisthesis. Significant progression of an associated spondylolisthesis is uncommon. There are data to indicate that sports participation does not increase the risk of progression of a low-grade slip [41]. When slip progression occurs, it is usually does so during the adolescent growth spurt, typically without any symptoms, and affected individuals need to be monitored radiographically through adolescence.

Studies in the general population have shown pars lesions to be a relatively common finding. Fredrickson and colleagues [25] prospectively studied 500 first-grade students with plain radiographs and found an overall

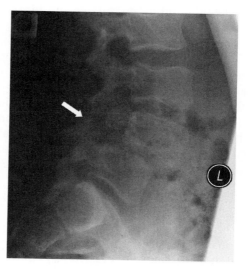

Fig. 1. Lateral radiograph of a young tennis player showing an isthmic spondylolisthesis with bilateral pars defects (*arrow*).

prevalence of spondylolysis of 4.4% at age 6 years. All of these lesions occurred without any symptoms. This number increased to 5.2% by age 12 years and to 6% by adulthood. Roche and Rowe [26] studied 4200 cadaveric spines and found an overall prevalence of 4.2%. The numbers are different in athletes, however, with large-scale studies of adolescent athletes showing rates of 8% to 14% [27,28]. Athletes participating in certain sports have much higher frequencies of spondylolysis than others. Some of the sports with the highest reported frequencies of pars lesions include gymnastics, weight lifting, throwing track and field sports, diving, wrestling, cricket, and crew [27,28,42–44]. Sports that involve frequent flexion/extension motions of the lumbar spine, particularly when combined with rotation, may place athletes at more risk for pars fractures.

History and physical examination can be helpful in establishing the diagnosis, although by definition, spinal imaging is essential. Symptomatic spondylolysis typically presents with axial LBP without radiation into the legs. The pain can come on acutely after a specific traumatic event (or even a relatively mundane event) or may progress gradually over time. The pain is usually worsened by activity and improves with rest. It is common to see the symptoms begin toward the end of one sports season, subside after the season, and then return when the athlete starts training for the next season. The pain can lateralize to the side of the lesion or be more generalized in the low back. Leg pain, paresthesias, or neurologic loss are not consistent with isolated spondylolysis and should suggest the presence of spondylolisthesis or other diagnoses in young athletes. There are no pathognomonic findings on physical examination for a pars lesion. The one-legged hyperextension maneuver (in which the patient stands on one leg and leans backward) has been proposed as a means of identifying the presence of a pars lesion, but a recent study on this test concluded that it was relatively unhelpful and had low sensitivity and specificity [45].

A number of diagnostic imaging modalities are available for evaluating the pars in an athlete who has suspected spondylolysis, and significant controversy exists regarding the optimal imaging strategy. Given the relatively high prevalence of asymptomatic pars lesions in adolescent athletes, it is not enough just to visualize a pars lesion. Ideally, the pars defect needs to be identified as the source of pain, and information on the potential for the lesion to heal should be obtained. In practical application, this means that multiple imaging studies are usually required to diagnose and treat athletes who have spondylolysis.

Plain radiography has been used in diagnosing pars lesions for some time and is the basis for diagnosis and follow-up in a large number of published studies. Nuclear imaging with bone scan with or without single-photon emission CT (SPECT), CT, and MRI have been shown to be more sensitive than plain radiography in the identification of pars lesions [46]. Typically, spondylolysis appears on plain radiographs as a lucency in the area of the pars (see Fig. 1). On oblique films, this lesion is characteristically described as a fracture "in the neck of the Scotty dog." In current use, the ability to identify and follow a spondylolisthesis may actually be the most important role of plain films in managing adolescents who have spondylolysis.

Radionuclide imaging, particularly SPECT, can be very helpful in the diagnostic evaluation of adolescent athletes who have LBP. Numerous studies have shown bone scan and SPECT to be more sensitive than plain radiography in the diagnosis of spondylolysis, and they appear to be superior to MRI and CT in this regard [47–54]. There are multiple studies that have shown that a positive bone scan or SPECT correlates with a symptomatic pars lesion [48,55–59], making SPECT a particularly useful screening tool in adolescent athletes who have LBP. A significant limitation in the use of radionuclide imaging, however, is specificity. Not all of the abnormalities seen in the posterior elements of adolescents on SPECT or bone scan represent pars lesions [46,50,52,60]. Additional imaging, particularly with CT, is generally required to clarify the bony abnormality in a patient who has a positive SPECT study (Fig. 2A, B and Fig. 3A).

Along with providing clarification of a bony process identified on nuclear imaging, CT can distinguish between well-corticated fracture margins (termed chronic lesions or nonunions by various investigators) and differing stages of more recent or incomplete fractures [46,54,60–62]. The stage of the pars lesion on CT has been found to be associated with the potential for bony healing [54,61]. Investigators have also identified a number of patients in whom there is increased activity in the area of the pars on SPECT but an incomplete fracture or no fracture noted on CT [42,52,54,60,62]. This finding seems most consistent with the presence of a stress reaction in the bone without overt fracture and speaks to the importance of correlating CT findings with nuclear imaging [60].

Although theoretically attractive, MRI currently has limitations as the primary imaging modality for adolescent athletes who have LBP. The advantages of MRI include the lack of ionizing radiation and the ability to identify disc abnormalities and other types of pathology. It can be difficult, however, to appreciate well the cortical detail at the pars on MRI. The important diagnostic findings on MRI in patients who have a potential pars lesion are those that are consistent with edema in the area of the pars or pedicle, suggestive of an acute fracture (see Fig. 3B). It is unfortunate that not much data exist on the clinical implications of these findings. Studies have shown significant limitations in the ability to identify and appropriately stratify pars lesions based on MRI, and it does not seem to be an effective screening tool as currently used [45,53]. A recent study comparing the relative utility of MRI compared with SPECT and CT found that MRI identified only 80% of the pars lesions seen on SPECT [45].

Overall, an adolescent athlete who has LBP and has signs or symptoms suggestive of a pars fracture should be assessed with limited plain films, particularly isolated standing anteroposterior and lateral views to identify a spondylolisthesis or gross bony abnormalities, followed by a SPECT study.

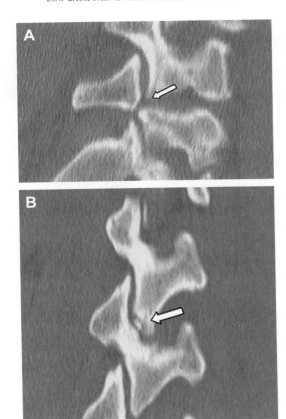

Fig. 2. CT oblique sagittal reformations. (*A*) A chronic pars lesion (*arrow*) with the classic appearance of a fracture in the "neck of the Scotty dog." (*B*) A lesion in the inferior articular process (*arrow*) in a young basketball player. A SPECT study of the same athlete had been interpreted as being consistent with spondylolysis.

If the SPECT study is positive, then a thin-cut CT (axial sequences of ≤1 mm thickness) should be obtained through the area of abnormality on SPECT to confirm the diagnosis and to stage the lesion for treatment. If the SPECT is negative, then it is highly unlikely that the athlete has a symptomatic pars defect, and other diagnoses should be considered.

In an era of evidence-based medicine, it is noteworthy that there are no controlled trials on the treatment of spondylolysis in adolescent athletes. A number of published case series have used a wide variety of treatment approaches. The essential element of care appears to be relative rest; however, the ideal extent of activity restriction involved and the length of time out of sports is unclear. Bracing is a particularly contentious issue in the management of spondylolysis. A number of investigators advocate the routine use of lumbosacral orthoses of various types in the management of these

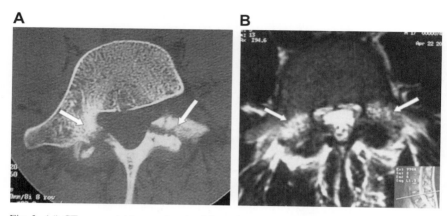

Fig. 3. (*A*) CT scan axial image showing bilateral pars fractures (*arrows*). (*B*) Corresponding T2-weighted axial MRI scan of the same patient showing hyperintense signal in the pedicles bilaterally (*arrows*) associated with the bilateral pars fractures. Note that the fractures are better appreciated on the CT image. (*From* Standaert CJ. The diagnosis and management of lumbar spondylolysis. Oper Tech Sports Med 2005;13(2):104; with permission.)

patients, whereas others do not. Biomechanical studies on the effects lumbosacral bracing show that bracing results in an increase in intervertebral motion at the lumbosacral junction in most individuals, and the main effect of bracing seems to be a restriction in gross body motion rather than restricting intersegmental mobility [63,64]. The results of outcome studies tend to be somewhat similar regarding rates of healing and return-to-play, regardless of the type or extent of bracing used, and studies have shown bony healing with the use of a rigid brace, a soft brace, and no brace [61,65–68]. There is also surprisingly little correlation between the extent of bony healing and return-to-play, with most studies addressing these issues showing relatively high rates of return-to-play and much lower rates of healing [62,67–70]. A recent study by Ruiz-Cotorro and colleagues [66] had the rare feature of including patients treated with a brace and patients treated without a brace. Although the numbers in this study were small, the investigators did not find any advantage for brace use in terms of achieving bony union.

Based on the current evidence, initial treatment for all athletes is rest, which ideally should include avoidance of all physical activity (particularly sports) beyond that needed for routine daily function. The duration of activity restriction is based on the patients' clinical response and the appearance of their pars lesion on CT. When the CT shows an early- or progressive-stage lesion, the athlete is advised to rest for 3 months. When the pars lesion has chronic features on CT, there is very little chance it will achieve a bony union, and rest is advised until the LBP has subsided [61]. Although preferred by some, the routine use of bracing is not uniformly supported in the literature. As a means of further restricting activity, a rigid brace may be used after 2 or 3 weeks of rest if symptoms are not resolving. After adequate rest for the stage of the lesion and restoration of pain-free range of motion, athletes can be placed into a comprehensive rehabilitation program. Generally, rehabilitation requires 2 to 4 months to complete, resulting in return to sport approximately 5 to 7 months after diagnosis in an athlete who has an acute pars lesion.

Surgical intervention is rarely required to treat the pain associated with spondylolysis. Potential indications for surgical intervention include progressive slip, intractable pain, the development of neurologic deficits, and segmental instability associated with pain. For patients who have a slip of 50% or greater, surgical treatment is usually considered the best option, and these patients should undergo surgical evaluation. There are a number of case series on athletes undergoing surgery for direct pars repair and returning to high-level sports, but return-to-play and long-term quality-of-life considerations need to be factored into decisions on surgical intervention.

As a routine issue, follow-up films are not necessary for patients who have a unilateral pars lesion without a spondylolisthesis who do well with conservative treatment. Those who have a spondylolisthesis need repeat plain films every 6 to 12 months while growing to monitor for possible slip progression, as do patients who have bilateral pars defects, particularly if very young at the time of presentation. Repeat imaging with CT can be helpful when it is necessary to determine the extent of healing or progression of the fracture. Additional diagnostic evaluation should also be considered in patients who are not responding well to what seems to be appropriate treatment.

Discogenic injuries

Discogenic LBP is a relatively uncommon but still significant problem in adolescent athletes. In their study of adolescents presenting to a sports medicine clinic with LBP compared with adults at a general orthopedic clinic, Micheli and Wood [38] attributed the LBP to disc abnormalities in about 50% of the adults but in only about 10% of the adolescents. In a series of 742 patients undergoing surgery for lumbar disc disease, adolescents (age <20 years) accounted for only 3.5% of the cases [71]. Disc abnormalities on imaging studies are less common in adolescents than in adults. In a study of 439 13-year-old children from the general population, about one third were noted to have discogenic abnormalities on MRI compared with over 50% of 40-year-olds in a similar study [72,73]. As noted previously, athletes in some sports have been found to have higher rates of degenerative disc changes than are seen in the general population [17,23]. Disc herniations in some young athletes may also be affected by genetic factors, and the rate of disc herniations occurring in individuals younger than 21 years is five times greater in those who have a positive family history [74].

Disc pathology can result in isolated LBP or radiating pain to the buttocks or lower extremities. The symptoms are generally worsened by activities involving flexion, rotation, or increases in intra-abdominal pressure; however, there are no true pathognomonic aspects of the history for discogenic pain. Similar symptoms can be seen with other types of spine pathology, and disc problems can present with other patterns of symptoms. Disc protrusions associated with congenital canal stenosis may represent somewhat of a distinct problem in athletes who have back or leg pain because there may be an increased risk of neurologic involvement and, potentially, a less favorable natural history [75]. These athletes may present with a history more consistent with spinal stenosis, including neurogenic claudication. As with all athletes who have low back disorders, a comprehensive physical examination including a neurologic evaluation is essential for appropriate treatment in those who have presumed discogenic abnormalities.

Treatment options for disc injuries in adolescent athletes are similar to those in adults, although there are a few distinct considerations regarding sports participation and age that may be relevant. Nonoperative care is clearly advised as the dominant form of treatment for most adolescent athletes who have discogenic pain [33,35,75,76]. A number of nonoperative treatment modalities are available for use, although there is limited study of their effectiveness in the adolescent population. These modalities include physical therapy to address lumbar stability and neuromuscular control, therapeutic modalities, manipulative care, massage, medications, and interventional care (eg, epidural injections). In general, it may be best to minimize the use of interventions and medications in this population, given some of the caveats mentioned previously regarding their use in adolescents. Surgical care is generally reserved for those who have (1) severe radicular pain not responding to optimal nonoperative care, (2) cauda equina involvement, or (3) progressive neurologic loss [35]. There also should be clear imaging and other diagnostic findings that correlate with the athlete's symptoms. In young athletes, there is a balance to be maintained between the long-term ramifications on global and spinal health and intervention to enhance performance. There are situations in which the athlete can live with pain or other restrictions but is limited in the performance of their sport. In some of these cases, surgery may enhance the ability of the athlete to perform. In others, surgery may address the underlying pathology but may not result in any meaningful improvement in sports performance while placing the athlete at risk for acute or long-term complications from intervention [75]. As with all other conditions, treatment for disc injuries needs to be directed toward the benefit of the whole individual.

Scheuermann's kyphosis

Scheuermann's kyphosis is a developmental condition of uncertain etiology affecting the thoracic or thoracolumbar spine and a relatively frequent cause of back pain in adolescents. The condition was originally described by Scheuermann in 1921 and is defined by the presence of anterior wedging of at least 5° in three consecutive vertebrae, end plate irregularities, disc space narrowing, and the presence of Schmorl's nodes (Fig. 4) [77,78]. The

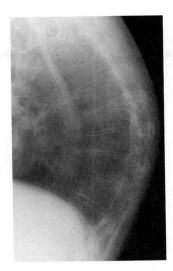

Fig. 4. A lateral radiograph showing the findings associated with Scheuermann's kyphosis. Note the multilevel vertebral body wedging, end plate irregularities, and disc height loss.

condition has an incidence reported to be 0.4% to 8.3% in the general population and may be more frequent in boys than in girls [77,78]. Some investigators have found the mean height in affected individuals to be greater than that in the overall population [78]. There have been a number of proposed etiologic factors, including mechanical injury, chronic anterior loading, osteoporosis, cartilage abnormalities, and various genetic factors; however, the precise cause or genetic basis of the disorder has not been elucidated [35,76,78].

Patients who have Scheuermann's kyphosis can present with pain, fatigue, or isolated complaints of deformity or poor posture. If present, the pain is usually in the area of the deformity and is worsened by activity. Neurologic symptoms or findings are rare. Patients typically present during adolescence; presentations before age 10 years are uncommon [35,76–78]. Physical examination is notable for postural changes associated with an increased thoracic kyphosis, including lumbar hyperlordosis and a forward head position. The kyphosis in Scheuermann's is rigid and does not typically correct with extension [78]. The natural history of the disorder is not well understood, but the symptoms often diminish as patients reach skeletal maturity. Adults who have a deformity of less than 60° have little chance of having back pain beyond that noted in the general population [76,78].

Treatment of Scheuermann's kyphosis depends on the extent of the symptoms and the degree of curvature. For patients who have a curve of less than 50° to 60°, flexibility and postural exercises may be helpful. Pain may respond to relative rest, anti-inflammatory medication, or bracing. For more substantial curves of 50° to 75° in a skeletally immature patient, bracing should be considered. For those who have even greater curves, bracing may not be helpful, and surgical treatment should be considered [76–78].

Although the kyphosis generally occurs in the thoracic spine, a less common lumbar variant of Scheuermann's has been described with end plate changes, Schmorl's nodes, and disc space narrowing, with less frequent vertebral wedging (Fig. 5). The lumbar variant is presumed to have a more clearly defined mechanical basis than typical Scheuermann's kyphosis and is seen in athletes participating in sports associated with rapid flexion/extension motions or with heavy lifting [35,76–78]. Although often thought of as simply a variant of thoracic Scheuermann's kyphosis, this condition may be a different clinical entity altogether [78]. Pain is typically located at the area of involvement in the thoracolumbar region and exacerbated by activity, particularly involving lumbar flexion. On examination, there is usually no marked kyphotic deformity, but there may be flattening of the lumbar lordosis. The natural history is typically nonprogressive, and treatment involves relative rest, anti-inflammatory medication, lumbar stabilization, flexibility and postural training, time, and occasionally the use of an orthosis [76–78].

Rehabilitation and return to play

A number of investigators have described rehabilitation programs for adolescent athletes who have various lumbar disorders, but there is surprisingly little in the way of formal study of this issue. Nonoperative rehabilitation programs tend to be somewhat empirically derived, and more research

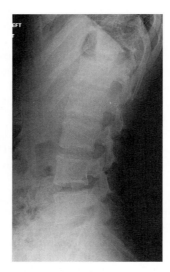

Fig. 5. A lateral radiograph showing the findings associated with the lumbar variant of Scheuermann's kyphosis. Note the end plate irregularities, disc height loss, Schmorl's nodes, and relative lack of vertebral body wedging.

into finite aspects of rehabilitation needs to be performed. This issue is complex, however, because nonoperative programs are multifactorial, and comprehensive rehabilitation generally addresses a number of factors affecting the injured athlete. In practical application, this approach means establishing an early and accurate diagnosis, initiating appropriate acute treatment of injured structures, performing a full assessment of the kinetic chain and athletic technique for factors that may be related to the primary injury, and identifying environmental or psychosocial barriers to performance. Given the available data, rehabilitation should progress through a structured, sport-specific program with a focus on specific motions, postures, and activities required in the performance of the athlete's chosen sport. Specific activities, timing, and progression of training in a given athlete depend heavily on the nature of any acute injury, on subsequent treatment, and on individual factors related to the athlete that affect performance [33,75,79].

Return to play after injury is allowed when the athlete has been given sufficient time to recover from his or her acute injury and has progressed through a sport-specific rehabilitation program. Return-to-play criteria include full, pain-free range of motion, appropriate aerobic conditioning, normal strength, and a demonstrated ability to perform sports-related skills without pain [80]. For low back injuries, athletes should also demonstrate adequate spinal awareness and dynamic postural control.

Summary

LBP is a common problem among young athletes. These individuals are at risk for significant structural injuries or nonmechanical problems that can be associated with their symptoms. Any athlete who has severe, persisting, or activity-limiting symptoms must be evaluated thoroughly. Clinicians must have a working knowledge of the developmental issues, injury patterns, and particular conditions that may affect a given athlete and be able to work with patients in addition to families, coaches, trainers, and others involved in the care and training of the injured athlete.

References

[1] Ferguson RL. Thoracic and lumbar spinal trauma of the immature spine. In: Herkowitz HN, Garfin SR, Eismont FJ, et al, editors. Rothman-Simeone the spine. 5th edition. Philadelphia: Saunders; 2006. p. 603–12.

[2] Clark P, Letts M. Trauma to the thoracic and lumbar spine in the adolescent. Can J Surg 2001;44(5):337–45.

[3] Commandre FA, Gagnerie G, Zakarian M, et al. The child, the spine and sport. J Sports Med Phys Fitness 1988;28(1):11–9.

[4] Cyron BM, Hutton WC. The fatigue strength of the lumbar neural arch in spondylolysis. J Bone Joint Surg Br 1978;60-B:234–8.

[5] Burton AK, Clarke RD, McClune TD, et al. The natural history of low back pain in adolescents. Spine 1996;21(20):2323–8.

[6] Harreby M, Nygaard B, Jessen T, et al. Risk factors for low back pain in a cohort of 1389 Danish school children: an epidemiologic study. Eur Spine J 1999;8(6):444–50.

[7] Kovacs FM, Gestoso M, Gil del Real MT, et al. Risk factors for non-specific low back pain in schoolchildren and their parents: a population based study. Pain 2003;103:239–68.

[8] Salminen JJ, Erkintalo M, Laine M, et al. Low back pain in the young. A prospective three-year follow-up study of subjects with and without low back pain. Spine 1995;20(19):2101–7.

[9] Taimela S, Kujala UM, Salminen JJ, et al. The prevalence of low back pain among children and adolescents: a nationwide, cohort-based questionnaire survey in Finland. Spine 1997; 22(10):1132–6.

[10] Troussier B, Davoine P, de Gaudemaris R, et al. Back pain in school children: a study among 1178 pupils. Scand J Rehabil Med 1994;26:143–6.

[11] Auvinen J, Tammelin T, Taimela S, et al. Associations of physical activity and inactivity with low back pain in adolescents. Scand J Med Sci Sports 2007 [epub ahead of print].

[12] Mogensen AM, Gausel AM, Wedderkopp N, et al. Is active participation in specific sport activities linked with back pain? Scand J Med Sci Sports 2007;17(6):680–6.

[13] Wedderkopp N, Leboeuf-Yde C, Andersen LB, et al. Back pain in children. No association with objectively measured level of physical activity. Spine 2003;28(17):2019–24.

[14] McBeth J, Jones K. Epidemiology of chronic musculoskeletal pain. Best Pract Res Clin Rheumatol 2007;21(3):403–25.

[15] Hestbaek L, Leboeuf-Yde C, Kyvik KO, et al. The course of low back pain from adolescence to adulthood: eight-year follow-up of 9600 twins. Spine 2006;31(4):468–72.

[16] Kujala UM, Taimela S, Erkintalo M, et al. Low back pain in adolescent athletes. Med Sci Sports Exerc 1996;28(2):165–70.

[17] Sward L, Hellstrom M, Jacobsson B, et al. Disc degeneration and associated abnormalities of the spine in elite gymnasts. A magnetic resonance imaging study. Spine 1991;16(4):437–43.

[18] Sward L, Hellstrom M, Jacobsson B, et al. Back pain and radiologic changes in the thoraco-lumbar spine of athletes. Spine 1990;15(2):124–9.

[19] Hickey GJ, Fricker PA, McDonald WA. Injuries to elite rowers over a 10-yr period. Med Sci Sports Exerc 1997;29(12):1567–72.

[20] Hosea TM, Gatt CJ. Back pain in golf. Clin Sports Med 1996;15(1):37–53.

[21] Iwamoto J, Abe H, Tsukimura Y, et al. Relationship between radiographic abnormalities of lumbar spine and incidence of low back pain in high school rugby players: a prospective study. Scand J Med Sci Sports 2005;15:163–8.

[22] Goldstein JD, Berger PE, Windler GE, et al. Spine injuries in gymnasts and swimmers: an epidemiologic investigation. Am J Sports Med 1991;19:463–8.

[23] Bennett DL, Nassar L, DeLano MC. Lumbar spine MRI in the elite-level female gymnast with low back pain. Skeletal Radiol 2006;35:503–9.

[24] Iwamoto J, Abe H, Tsukimura Y, et al. Relationship between radiographic abnormalities of lumbar spine and incidence of low back pain in high school and college football players. Am J Sports Med 2004;32(3):781–6.

[25] Fredrickson BE, Baker D, McHolick WJ, et al. The natural history of spondylolysis and spondylolisthesis. J Bone Joint Surg Am 1984;66:699–707.

[26] Roche MA, Rowe GG. The incidence of separate neural arch and coincident bone variations: a survey of 4,200 skeletons. Anat Rec 1951;109:233–52.

[27] Rossi F, Dragoni S. The prevalence of spondylolysis and spondylolisthesis in symptomatic elite athletes: radiographic findings. Radiography 2001;7:37–42.

[28] Soler T, Calderon C. The prevalence of spondylolysis in the Spanish elite athlete. Am J Sports Med 2000;28:57–62.

[29] Lundin O, Hellstrom M, Nilsson I, et al. Back pain and radiologic changes in the thoraco-lumbar spine of athletes: a long-term follow-up. Scand J Med Sci Sports 2001;11: 103–9.

[30] Teitz CC, O'Kane JW, Lind BK. Back pain in former intercollegiate rowers: a long-term follow-up study. Am J Sports Med 2003;31(4):590–5.

[31] Tsai L, Wredmark T. Spinal posture, sagittal mobility, and subjective rating of back problems in former female elite gymnasts. Spine 1993;18:872–5.

[32] Anderson SJ. Assessment and management of the pediatric and adolescent patient with low back pain. Phys Med Rehabil Clin N Am 1991;2(1):157–85.

[33] Bono CM. Low-back pain in athletes. J Bone Joint Surg Am 2004;86:382–96.

[34] Hosalkar H, Dormans J. Back pain in children requires extensive workup. Biomechanics 2003;10(6):51–8.

[35] Mason DE. Back pain in children. Pediatr Ann 1999;28(12):727–38.

[36] Standaert CJ, Herring SA, Cole AJ, et al. The lumbar spine and sports. In: Cole AJ, Herring SA, editors. The low back pain handbook. 2nd edition. Philadelphia: Hanley & Belfus; 2003. p. 385–404.

[37] Dodge TL, Jaccard JJ. The effect of high school sports participation on the use of performance-enhancing substances in young adulthood. J Adolesc Health 2006;39:367–73.

[38] Micheli LJ, Wood R. Back pain in young athletes: significant differences from adults in causes and patterns. Arch Pediatr Adolesc Med 1995;149:15–8.

[39] Wiltse LL, Newman PH, Macnab I. Classification of spondylolysis and spondylolisthesis. Clin Orthop Relat Res 1976;117:23–9.

[40] Wiltse LL, Widell EH, Jackson DW. Fatigue fracture: the basic lesion in isthmic spondylolisthesis. J Bone Joint Surg Am 1975;57:17–22.

[41] Muschik M, Hahnel H, Robinson PN, et al. Competitive sports and the progression of spondylolisthesis. J Pediatr Orthop 1996;16:364–9.

[42] Gregory PL, Batt ME, Kerslake RW. Comparing spondylolysis in cricketers and soccer players. Br J Sports Med 2004;38:737–42.

[43] McCarroll JR, Miller JM, et al. Lumbar spondylolysis and spondylolisthesis in college football players: a prospective study. Am J Sports Med 1986;14:404–6.

[44] Semon RL, Spengler D. Significance of lumbar spondylolysis in college football players. Spine 1981;6:172–4.

[45] Masci L, Pike J, Malara F, et al. Use of the one-legged hyperextension test and magnetic resonance imaging in the diagnosis of active spondylolysis. Br J Sports Med 2006;40:940–6.

[46] Harvey CJ, Richenberg JL, Saifuddin A, et al. Pictorial review: the radiological investigation of lumbar spondylolysis. Clin Radiol 1998;53:723–8.

[47] Jackson DW, Wiltse LL, Dingeman RD, et al. Stress reactions involving the pars interarticularis in young athletes. Am J Sports Med 1981;9:304–12.

[48] Elliott S, Hutson MA, Wastie ML. Bone scintigraphy in the assessment of spondylolysis in patients attending a sports injury clinic. Clin Radiol 1988;39:269–72.

[49] Anderson K, Sarwark JF, Conway JJ, et al. Quantitative assessment with SPECT imaging of stress injuries of the pars interarticularis and response to bracing. J Pediatr Orthop 2000;20: 28–33.

[50] Bellah RD, Summerville DA, Treves ST, et al. Low back pain in adolescent athletes: detection of stress injury to the pars interarticularis with SPECT. Radiology 1991;180:509–12.

[51] Bodner RJ, Heyman S, Drummond DS, et al. The use of single photon emission computed tomography (SPECT) in the diagnosis of low back pain in young patients. Spine 1988;3:1155–60.

[52] Congeni J, McCulloch J, Swanson K. Lumbar spondylolysis: a study of natural progression in athletes. Am J Sports Med 1997;25:248–53.

[53] Campbell RSD, Grainger AJ, Hide IG, et al. Juvenile spondylolysis: a comparative analysis of CT, SPECT, and MRI. Skeletal Radiol 2005;34:63–73.

[54] Stretch RA, Botha T, Chandler S, et al. Back injuries in young fast bowlers—a radiologic investigation of the healing of spondylolysis and pedicle sclerosis. S Afr Med J 2003;93:611–6.

[55] Lowe J, Schachner E, Hirschberg E, et al. Significance of bone scintigraphy in symptomatic spondylolysis. Spine 1984;9:653–5.

[56] Collier BD, Johnson RP, Carrera GF, et al. Painful spondylolysis or spondylolisthesis studied by radiography and single photon emission computed tomography. Radiology 1985;154:207–11.

[57] Itoh K, Hashimoto T, Shigenobu K, et al. Bone SPECT of symptomatic lumbar spondylolysis. Nucl Med Commun 1996;17:389–96.

[58] Lusins JO, Elting JJ, Cicoria AD, et al. SPECT evaluation of lumbar spondylolysis and spondylolisthesis. Spine 1994;19:608–12.

[59] Raby N, Mathews S. Symptomatic spondylolysis: correlation of CT and SPECT with clinical outcome. Clin Radiol 1993;48:97–9.

[60] Gregory PL, Batt ME, Kerslake RW, et al. The value of combining single photon emission computerised tomography and computerised tomography in the investigation of spondylolysis. Eur Spine J 2004;13:503–9.

[61] Fujii K, Katoh S, Sairyo K, et al. Union of defects in the pars interarticularis of the lumbar spine in children and adolescents: the radiologic outcome after conservative treatment. J Bone Joint Surg Br 2004;86:225–31.

[62] Miller SF, Congeni J, Swanson K. Long-term functional and anatomical follow-up of early detected spondylolysis in young athletes. Am J Sports Med 2004;32:928–33.

[63] Axelsson P, Johnsson R, Stromqvist B. Effect of lumbar orthosis on intervertebral mobility. Spine 1992;17:678–81.

[64] Calmels P, Fayolle-Minon I. An update on orthotic devices for the lumbar spine based on a review of the literature. Rev Rhum Engl Ed 1996;63:285–91.

[65] Standaert CJ, Herring SA. Spondylolysis: a critical review. Br J Sports Med 2000;34:415–22.

[66] Ruiz-Cotorro A, Balius-Matas R, Estruch-Massana AE, et al. Spondylolysis in young tennis players. Br J Sports Med 2006;40:441–6.

[67] Steiner ME, Micheli LJ. Treatment of symptomatic spondylolysis and spondylolisthesis with the modified Boston brace. Spine 1985;10:937–43.

[68] Blanda J, Bethem D, Moats W, et al. Defects of pars interarticularis in athletes: a protocol for nonoperative treatment. J Spinal Disord 1993;6:406–11.

[69] Iwamoto J, Takeda T, Wakano K. Returning athletes with severe low back pain and spondylolysis to original sporting activities with conservative treatment. Scand J Med Sci Sports 2004;14:346–51.

[70] Sys J, Michielsen J, Bracke P, et al. Nonoperative treatment of active spondylolysis in elite athletes with normal X-ray findings: literature review and results of conservative treatment. Eur Spine J 2001;10:498–504.

[71] Kumar R, Kumar V, Das NK, et al. Adolescent lumbar disc disease: findings and outcome. Childs Nerv Syst 2007;23(11):1295–9.

[72] Kjaer P, Leboeuf-Yde C, Sorensen JS, et al. An epidemiologic study of MRI and low back pain in 13-year-old children. Spine 2005;30(7):798–806.

[73] Kjaer P, Leboeuf-Yde C, Korsholm L, et al. Magnetic resonance imaging and low back pain in adults: a diagnostic imaging study of 40 year-old men and women. Spine 2005;30(10):1173–80.

[74] Ala-Kokko L. Genetic risk factors for lumbar disc disease. Ann Med 2002;34:42–7.

[75] Watkins RG. Lumbar disc injury in the athlete. Clin Sports Med 2002;21(1):147–65.

[76] Waicus KM, Smith BW. Back injuries in the pediatric athlete. Curr Sports Med Rep 2002;1:52–8.

[77] Karol LA. Back pain in children and adolescents. In: Herkowitz HN, Garfin SR, Eismont FJ, et al, editors. Rothman-Simeone the spine. 5th edition. Philadelphia: Saunders; 2006. p. 493–506.

[78] Shah SWA, Takemitsu M, Westerlund LE, et al. Pediatric kyphosis: Scheuermann's disease and congenital deformity. In: Herkowitz HN, Garfin SR, Eismont FJ, et al, editors. Rothman-Simeone the spine. 5th edition. Philadelphia: Saunders; 2006. p. 565–85.

[79] Standaert CJ, Herring SA, Pratt TW. Rehabilitation of the athlete with low back pain. Curr Sports Med Rep 2004;3(1):35–40.

[80] Herring SA, Kibler WB. A framework for rehabilitation. In: Kibler WB, Herring SA, Press JM, et al, editors. Functional rehabilitation of sports and musculoskeletal injuries. Gaithersburg (MD): Aspen; 1998. p. 1–8.

PHYSICAL MEDICINE
AND REHABILITATION
CLINICS OF
NORTH AMERICA

ELSEVIER
SAUNDERS

Phys Med Rehabil Clin N Am
19 (2008) 305–318

Examination and Treatment of Pediatric Injuries of the Hip and Pelvis

Brandee L. Waite, MD[a],*, Brian J. Krabak, MD, MBA[b]

[a]Department of Physical Medicine and Rehabilitation, University of California
Davis School of Medicine, 4860 Y Street, Suite 3850, Sacramento, CA 95817, USA
[b]Department of Physical Medicine and Rehabilitation, University of Washington
School of Medicine, 4245 Roosevelt Way 354740, Seattle, WA 98105, USA

Injuries to the hip and pelvis are the least common of lower extremity injuries in youth sports, but include many of the more serious conditions [1]. This article describes the bone and soft-tissue conditions of the hip and pelvis that may present to health care providers caring for the pediatric and adolescent sporting population. The article discusses epidemiology, mechanisms, clinical presentation, evaluation, and treatment options.

Bone development of the hip

The acetabulum and femur start development intrauterine at 6 weeks [2]. The acetabulum begins as a shallow depression from bony precursor cells that eventually form the pubis, ilium, and schium of the pelvis. Other cells grow to start the formation of the proximal, central, and distal aspects of the femur. By week 8, the primary ossification centers of the femur appear with development of the surrounding soft tissue and internal rotation of the limb. At this time, development begins in the arterial supply of the proximal femur. By 12 to 14 weeks, the acetabulum develops a series of blood vessels while a network of vessels forms around the femoral neck. Hip growth and maturation continue for the next 20 weeks.

After birth, the acetabulum and femur undergo formation of secondary ossification centers at different stages. Initially, the acetabular bone is a cartilaginous complex that eventually forms ossification centers by age 8 to 9 years [3]. The femoral shaft ossification center starts developing during the first year of life. During the first 3 years, the femoral head is slightly

---

* Corresponding author.
E-mail address: brandee.waite@ucdmc.ucdavis.edu (B.L. Waite).

1047-9651/08/$ - see front matter © 2008 Elsevier Inc. All rights reserved.
doi:10.1016/j.pmr.2007.12.005

larger in its anterior-posterior length than in its transverse length. However, by age 3, it will become more spherical in nature. From birth to eventual physeal closure, the blood supply will be limited by the ability of the various vessels to supply the femoral head across the growth plate.

Throughout childhood and early adolescence, the underlying acetabulum, femoral bone, and pelvis continue to develop. Various apophyses appear, mostly occurring from ages 13 to 15 years (Table 1). During this time, the underlying bone is weaker at the apophyseal joint compared with the surrounding tendons, ligaments, and muscles. Any excessive contraction of the muscles or stretching on the ligaments is more likely to lead to separation of the apophysis rather than tearing of the tendon or muscle [4]. Fusion of the femoral complex and acetabulum with the ilium, ischium, and pubis is mostly completed by 16 to 18 years of age.

Bone conditions

Apophyseal injuries: anterior inferior iliac spine, iliac crest

Apophyseal avulsion injuries occur in skeletally immature athletes because of the inherent weakness across the open apophysis [5]. Incidence is increasing, especially in the 14- to 17-year-old age group as a result of increased participation in competitive sports [6]. An apophysis is a bony growth center (physis) where tendon attaches to bone. Until skeletal maturation is reached, the tendon attached to the site is stronger than the connection between the apophysis and the underlying bone [4]. Because of this biomechanical weakness, forceful contraction of the muscle results in separation of the epiphyseal plate (referred to as an avulsion fracture). Once the skeleton is mature, the physes are fused and thus stronger than the muscle or tendon, making apophyseal injuries obsolete. The same muscle contraction that causes apophyseal avulsion in adolescents causes tendon or muscle tears in adults. Though avulsion fractures can occur at any major muscle attachment, the most common sites are the sartorius attachment at the

Table 1
Age of appearance and fusion of apophyses in hip and pelvis

Apophysis	Appearance (y)	Fusion (y)	Related muscle group(s)
AIIS	13–15	16–18	Quadriceps
ASIS	13–15	21–25	Sartorious
Lesser trochanter	11–12	16–17	Iliopsoas
Greater trochanter	2–3	16–17	Gluteal
Ischial tuberosity	13–15	20–25	Hamstrings
Iliac crest	13–15	21–25	Abdominal obliques
			Latissimus dorsi

Abbreviations: AIIS, anterior inferior iliac spine; ASIS, anterior superior iliac spine.
From Anderson SJ. Lower extremity injuries in youth sports. Pediatr Clin North Am 2002;49(3):627–41; with permission.

anterior superior iliac spine, the rectus femoris attachment at the anterior inferior iliac spine, and the hamstring attachment at the ischial tuberosity.

Patients present with a history of activity-induced acute-onset pain, often accompanied with an audible pop or snap [4]. The injuries often occur during sports involving explosive or burst types of movement, such as American football, dance, soccer, and gymnastics. The patient characteristically assumes a position that minimizes stretch of the associated muscle [6]. Physical examination reveals tenderness and possibly swelling at the region overlying the apophysis, pain with passive stretch of the associated muscle group, and often pain with resisted contraction of the affected muscle.

Plain radiographs show a pathologic widening of the physis and the avulsed bone. Though the diagnosis is often made clinically, radiographs are helpful in determining the size of the avulsed fragment and the degree of bony displacement [6]. Treatment includes rest, ice, and protected weight-bearing with crutches for pain-free ambulation. Casting or bracing is not needed. Once the patient can ambulate without pain, a simple program of therapeutic exercise with a goal of stretching and strengthening the affected muscles. Low-impact activities, such as cycling, elliptic training, and swimming, can be initiated at this time as well. This is followed by a gradual return to running with progression to cutting, sprinting, and jumping [4]. Once these activities can be done without pain in a controlled environment, the patient can return to practice and eventually to competition. Follow-up radiographs are not required unless symptoms continue to limit activities. Surgical intervention is rare and is reserved for cases with significant ongoing symptoms. Surgery may also be indicated when there is a large fragment with greater than 2-cm displacement, though optimal timing for surgical intervention remains debatable [6]. There are no significant potential complications other than prolonged healing time and persistent symptoms.

Hip dislocation

Pediatric hip dislocation is relatively rare. Most cases are posterior dislocations. Low-energy dislocations (resulting from sporting or playing activities or from a fall from less than 10 ft) account for roughly 65% of posterior pediatric hip dislocations, with high-energy dislocations (resulting from a motor vehicle accident or fall from greater than 10 ft) accounting for the remaining 35% [7]. Posterior dislocations can occur when someone falls on top of a kneeling player [8].

Standard radiographs are the preferred initial imaging studies. Additionally, CT scan can be done to evaluate for fracture not seen on radiograph if there is high clinical suspicion or in cases where there is persistent or suspected posterior joint instability [9].

Closed reduction under conscious sedation or, less commonly, general anesthesia is the initial treatment. Occasionally, additional open reduction may be indicated if there are associated intra-articular fracture fragments or interposed soft tissue [7]. After a closed reduction, traction followed by mobilization and protected weight-bearing with crutches for 6 weeks is often used. An alternative postreduction course involves 6 weeks of using a spica cast followed by protected weight-bearing with crutches [7]. Physical therapy may be prescribed to focus initially on range of motion, progressing to strengthening and gait-training as weight-bearing restrictions are removed.

The vast majority of patients have full recovery without residual pain or limitation in sporting activities. Some experience mild aching with changes in the weather or a mild limp. Very few have moderate or severe pain or limp (approximately 5%) [7]. In a retrospective study of pediatric hip dislocations [7], the most common complications were associated fractures (17%) and avascular necrosis (12%). Associated fractures can include the posterior wall acetabulum or femoral head osteochondral, and occur almost exclusively in high-energy dislocations. Avascular necrosis of the femoral head can become evident on radiographs as soon as 2 months following dislocation. It is associated with prolonged time to reduction (greater than 6 hours) and does not appear to be associated with patient age, energy level of the dislocation, or the associated fracture. Persistent asymmetry postreduction can be due to soft-tissue interposition of a torn labrum, including lateral acetabular apophysis trapped within the joint [9]. Other potential complications include coxa magna, heterotopic ossification, and recurrent dislocation.

Legg-Calvé-Perthes disease

Legg-Calvé-Perthes disease comes on in the first decade, predominates in boys ages 4 to 8 years, and has a male/female ratio of 5:15 [5]. Bilateral cases occur in 8% to 24% of cases [5]. Literature is conflicting on potential causes of Legg-Calvé-Perthes disease. Most agree that the predominant cause is hypovascularity due to repetitive vascular injuries, though the underlying mechanism causing vascular insufficiency is still debated. Hypotheses center on thrombophillic mechanisms or transient elevations in intracapsular pressure. Pathology of this disease is complex, involving idiopathic self-limiting avascular necrosis of the femoral head [6]. Following the necrosis, there is resorption, collapse, and subsequent remodeling repair. More complete remodeling, which can be influenced with treatment, occurs more often in children with earlier presentation because of greater time for growth and remodeling before reaching skeletal maturity [5].

Patients present with insidious-onset painless limp, usually affecting only one leg. If pain is present, it is usually mild, exacerbated with exercise, and often referred to the knee [6]. Limitations of internal rotation and abduction are seen on physical examination. These limitations can be caused by either muscle spasm or synovitis in early stages and by bony impingement in later stages [6].

There are several classification systems used. Most widely used is the Herring lateral pillar classification system, which uses anteroposterior radiographs to determine the degree of involvement of the lateral portion of the femoral head. Group A hips have no involvement of the lateral pillar, meaning no density changes or loss of height in the lateral third of the femoral head (lateral pillar). Group B hips have some lucency in the lateral pillar and up to 50% of height loss. Group C hips have more lucency and greater than 50% height loss [10]. The Stulberg classification uses the shape of the femoral head to delineate between groups. Class I hips are normal. Class II hips have spherical, larger than normal femoral heads, shorter femoral necks, or abnormally steep acetabulae. Class III hips have heads that are nonspherical (ovoid, mushroom-shaped, or umbrella-shaped) but not flat. Class IV hips have flat heads and acetabulae [11]. The Caterall classification based on percent involvement of the epiphysis (25%, 50%, 75%, or 100%) is now infrequently used.

Plain radiographs are usually sufficient for diagnosis (Fig. 1). Treatment can be nonoperative (bracing) or operative (osteotomy). A large multicenter study [12] has shown that in children up to 8 years of age who present with lateral pillar group B hips have similar favorable outcomes whether treated operatively or nonoperatively. However, children over 8 years old with presentation in group B or B/C border had statistically significantly improved outcomes with surgery than with nonoperative management. Children who presented in the lateral pillar C classification had poorer outcomes regardless of age or treatment.

Osteitis pubis

Osteitis pubis is not commonly seen in young children, but may be seen in late-adolescent runners, late-adolescent soccer players, and young women

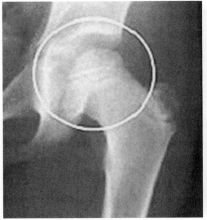
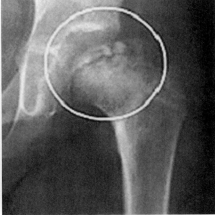

Normal hip   **Hip with perthes**

Fig. 1. Radiograph of hip with Legg-Calvé-Perthes disease. (*From* Children's Specialists of San Diego. Legg-Calves-Perthes disease. Available at: http://www.cssd.us/body.cfm?id=513. Accessed January 21, 2008; with permission.)

during pregnancy. It is one of the most common causes of chronic groin pain in the athletic population [13]. There is a reported incidence of 0.5% to 0.7% in the overall athletic population [14], but there are no reports specifically on pediatric incidence. It is most commonly seen in adults age 30 to 40. Pain at the pubic symphysis is the hallmark of osteitis pubis. It is an aseptic inflammatory condition that can cause erosion and sclerosis at the joint margins [15]. The most likely mechanism is repetitive stress from shearing forces at the joint or from traction of pelvic musculature [16]. Limited hip or sacroiliac range of motion may contribute to increased stresses at the pubic symphysis as well [17].

Patients present with complaint of insidious-onset, activity-related pain in the groin, anterior hip, or low abdomen. Male patients may have referred scrotal pain. Most do not note pain specifically at the pubic symphysis. However, they are quite tender to palpation over the joint. Pain may also be provoked by resisted active adduction if the distal symphysis is involved, or by sit-ups if the proximal symphysis is involved [17].

Plain radiographs are frequently normal in early or mild cases, but may show widening of the symphysis, irregular contour, or sclerosis in more advanced cases. In pediatric cases, radiographic abnormalities at the pubic symphysis may be difficult to distinguish from normal developmental ossification. Bone scan may show increased radioisotope uptake, but some symptomatic patients may not show abnormalities. MRI, which is increasingly used for definitive diagnosis, can show marrow edema in early stages or low signal on both T1 and T2 images in later stages [18].

This condition is usually a self-limited process, but some patients have a prolonged healing course, taking more than a year for complete resolution. Symptoms may be modified with use of oral anti-inflammatory medications or physical therapy aimed at stretching the adductors and improving hip range of motion. Correction of any biomechanical abnormalities that cause increased stress at the symphysis should be addressed in therapy as well. Any notable leg-length discrepancy should be corrected with a heel wedge or orthotics. In selected patients, fluoroscopy-guided diagnostic/therapeutic steroid and anesthetic injection may be used to confirm and treat the condition [15]. However, in the pediatric population, injection should be considered only after conservative measures have been exhausted. Some adults with persistent symptoms go on to have surgical interventions, but there is no literature recommending this type of intervention in children. Other than chronic pain in persistent cases, no significant complications of osteitis pubis are known.

Slipped capital femoral epiphysis

Slipped capital femoral epiphysis (SCFE) is an acquired separation of the proximal femoral head (epiphysis) from the remainder of the femur through the growth plate [19]. A query of a national pediatric database [20] found the incidence to be 10.80 for every 100,000 children with average age of onset of 12.7 years for boys and 11.2 years for girls, with overall male/female ratio of 1.65:1. Incidence was higher in black, Native American, Latino, and Asian/Pacific Islander children than in white children. Bilateral SCFE occurs in roughly 25% to 40% of cases [21].

The condition is caused when greater shearing stress is applied to the femoral head than can be tolerated by the open physis. It is usually associated with local trauma and may be mediated by other factors, including obesity and endocrine disorders [19]. Children present with pain in the hip, groin, thigh, or, occasionally, the knee (due to sensory distribution of the obturator and femoral nerves) [19]. History of trauma may or may not be noted predating pain or limping gait. Most will be able to bear weight, but may have an abnormal gait. Classic physical examination finding is external rotation and abduction of the hip when testing hip flexion in a supine patient [22]. In chronic cases, there may be mild disuse atrophy of the thigh and gluteal muscles. In cases of unstable SCFE, there is specific history of injury or fall leading to pain and inability to bear weight on the affected limb.

SCFE is considered stable if the child can ambulate and unstable if the child cannot tolerate even crutch-assisted ambulation. Radiographic classification can be made on the amount of slippage. Up to 32% slippage or up to 30° slip angle is considered mild; 33% to 50% slippage or 30° to 60° slip angle is moderate; and greater than 50% slippage or greater than 60° slip angle is severe. Clinical classification includes acute (symptoms less than 3 weeks), chronic (symptoms greater than 3 weeks), or acute on chronic (recent exacerbation of previous symptoms lasting more than 3 weeks.)

Anteroposterior and frog-leg views of the pelvis can help confirm diagnosis, though frog-leg position should be avoided when an unstable slip is suspected (Fig. 2). In cases with high clinical suspicion and normal radiographs, MRI can detect edema or other abnormality of the physis [23]. Non–weight-bearing restrictions (crutches or wheelchair) should be instituted as soon as SCFE is suspected to avoid potentiating further slippage. Stable slips are treated electively with in situ percutaneous pinning (minimally invasive with fluoroscopic guidance). Postoperatively, 6 to 8 weeks of limited or non–weight-bearing status is required. Unstable or severe slips usually require an open procedure, possibly corrective osteotomy. Because of the fairly frequent rate of bilateral SCFE, the contralateral hip should be monitored until skeletal maturity is reached.

Early diagnosis and treatment are key to avoiding potential prolonged morbidity. Avascular necrosis of the femoral head is the most serious potential complication, and occurs most often in severe or unstable cases. Chondrolysis (acute cartilage necrosis) occurs in 5% to 7% of SCFE cases [24] and, if not self-limited, can progress to severe pain and contracture, requiring arthrodesis [19]. Other potential complications include loss of motion, pain, and arthrosis [20]. More severe or untreated cases can lead to altered

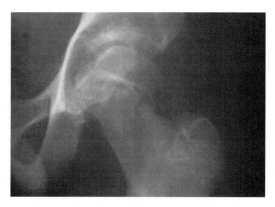

Fig. 2. Radiograph of hip with slipped capital femoral epiphysis. (*From* Wheeless CR. Wheeless' textbook of orthopaedics. Brooklandville, MD: Data Trace Publishing, 2007; with permission. Copyright © 2007 Data Trace Publishing Co. All rights reserved. www.wheelessonline.com.

hip mechanics, causing early degenerative change, potentially leading to need for total hip arthroplasty at an early age.

Stress fractures: femoral neck, pubic ramus, sacral

Stress fractures in young athletes usually stem from one or more of the following: relative osteoporosis due to nutritional or hormonal imbalances, inadequate muscle strength or endurance to provide maximum shock absorption during impact activities, changes in footwear or running surface, or acute increases in training regimen [17]. The most common sites for children are the tibia, fibula, and pars interarticularis of the lumbar spine. These combined account for approximately 85% of pediatric stress fractures [8]. Stress fractures in the hip region are much less common and can occur in the femoral neck, pubic ramus, and sacrum. These types of fractures are also seen in adult athletes, and more commonly in the elderly with osteoporosis.

In children, adolescents, and young adults, stress fractures are related to trabecular inability to withstand increased stresses applied to the area over time [25]. Contributing mechanisms include repetitive overload and impact, abnormal stress distribution from continued activity in the presence of muscle fatigue, and change in ground reaction force (altering the stress pattern in the bone) [26]. These are considered to be fatigue fractures in the adolescent population, in contrast to the insufficiency fractures seen in the elderly with suboptimal bone mass to withstand normal physiologic stress [27].

The location of the stress fracture determines the clinical presentation. Femoral neck and pubic ramus lesions cause groin or anterior thigh pain; sacral lesions cause lower back or gluteal pain [17,28]. Physical examination may show limited painful internal rotation or pain with hopping on the affected leg in femoral neck or pubic ramus stress fractures. Pain may be difficult to localize in femoral neck fractures, but tenderness with direct palpation over the pubic ramus is common. In sacral stress fractures, in addition to pain with hopping, patients may have paramedian tenderness on one side of the sacrum or at the sacroiliac joint, positive flamingo test (pain with single-leg stance on the affected side), or positive FABER maneuver (flexion, abduction, external rotation of the hip) [28].

Abnormalities on plain radiographs may be absent or mild and frequently lag behind symptoms by a month or more. They are usually insufficient to detect sacral stress fractures [28]. Bone scintigraphy can help make early diagnosis, but isotope uptake in the sacral region may be attributed to sacroiliac pathology rather than stress fracture. CT scan and MRI are more specific and are the imaging studies of choice. CT scan can help stage the fracture line and gives better imaging of the bony morphology, while MRI has the benefit of imaging without ionizing radiation [28].

Femoral neck stress fractures can be superior (traction/tension side) or inferior (compression side). Due to the high risk of progression, superior femoral neck stress fractures are treated surgically with open reduction and internal fixation. The other types of stress fractures mentioned here usually respond to relative rest for 6 to 12 weeks with a gradual return to sport after symptoms resolve. Treatment should also aim to address and modify risk factors. Maintenance of appropriate hormonal and nutritional balance, modification of training (eg, intensity, duration, surface), and modification of footwear can help reduce recurrences [17]. Stress fractures at the traction/tension location have high risk of progressing to complete fracture with associated complications of potential displacement and avascular necrosis [17]. Lesions on the compression side, pubic ramus, and sacrum have low risk of progression.

Soft tissue

Hip pointer (iliac crest contusion)

Though actual incidence is not reported in the literature, hip pointer is a common injury in rugby, American football, and other collision or tackling sports. The cause of a hip pointer is a direct blow to the iliac crest. It can therefore be both a bone and soft-tissue injury as it can cause bruising to both the iliac crest and the overlying soft tissue. Occasionally, the term is incorrectly used with injuries to the musculature around the hip resulting from bending or twisting movements. However, correct use of the sports medical terminology restricts the diagnosis to contusion caused by a direct blow. It is usually caused by an opponent's knee, head, or shoulder, while ill-fitting or inadequate hip pads may be a contributing factor [29].

Patients will report a history of a blow to the hip, or of being tackled without recollection of the direct blow. They have significant pain with movements, particularly sneezing, coughing, or running and are exquisitely tender to palpation of the iliac crest [29]. There is frequently swelling or bruising as well.

Plain radiographs are used to rule out an associated fracture. Icing, rest, and anti-inflammatory pain medications may be used to modify symptoms. As with most contusions, hip pointers are self-limited and resolve with time, depending on the severity of the blow. Once swelling and pain have decreased, therapeutic exercises may be initiated with a goal of restoring strength and flexibility to regional muscles [4]. Patients can gradually return to sports as tolerated, with attention to proper equipment and technique to prevent future injuries. There are no significant complications other than acute pain and possible pain-related disability.

Muscle strains and tears: adductor, quadriceps, hamstrings

Strain is a general term applied to muscle injuries. Adductor strain is the most common cause of groin pain in athletes [17]. In soccer players, rates as high as 10% to 18% have been reported [30,31]. Muscle strain, with or without associated tearing, is the most common athletic injury. In addition to the adductor, hip strains can affect iliopsoas, quadriceps, and hamstring muscles. Tears can occur in the muscle belly, though they are more common at the musculotendinous junction, where the well-vascularized muscle belly transitions to the poorly vascularized tendon.

Sudden forceful contraction (eccentric or concentric), quick midmovement directional change, falls, and persistent activity with muscle fatigue (undertraining or overuse) can all cause muscle strains and tears. Direct blows usually cause contusions rather than strains or tears, though a blow can cause an athlete to fall or make a directional change that then leads to a strain. Biomechanical abnormalities (eg, leg-length discrepancy, motion abnormalities, muscle imbalances) may also be contributing factors.

Patients may present with or without history of an acute accident or incident that preceded pain. They almost always report pain with activities using the affected muscle (eg, walking, standing from sitting position, sitting from standing position). On physical examination, they have pain with palpation and resisted muscle contraction [30]. It is important to rule out other causes of similar pain, such as osteitis pubis or sports hernia [17].

Strains can be classified as mild, moderate, or severe. Tears can be complete or incomplete. Diagnosis is made clinically. However, radiographs can be used to exclude associated fractures or avulsions [30]. Ultrasound can be used to diagnose tears, but not strains [18]. MRI can be used to confirm strains or tears, but is generally not needed unless there is significant pain or limitation in function.

Initial treatment of acute strains and partial tears includes icing, rest, and oral anti-inflammatory medications for pain management. Strains and partial tears to the muscle belly usually resolve after a period of relative rest, with return to sport accompanied by appropriate strength and flexibility training. Injuries to the musculotendinous junction likely require more aggressive formal physical therapy and rehabilitation after a period of adequate rest. In patients with persistent function-limiting adductor longus strain, surgical tenotomy may be indicated. Complete tears through the tendon or at the bony insertion are rare and tend to do better with surgical repair [32]. Strains may progress to partial tears, and partial tears to complete tears if the athlete returns to sports and activities without adequate time for healing or appropriate strength and flexibility rehabilitation training.

Snapping hip

Also known as coxa saltans, snapping hip is characterized by palpable or audible snapping that occurs with specific hip movements (described later) [33]. This disorder occurs most often in 15- to 40-year-olds [34]. It is more prevalent in women, particularly ballet dancers. Some literature reports up to 90% of ballet dancers have experienced snapping hip [35]. There are three causes of snapping: external, internal, and intra-articular pathology. The external type is most common and is caused by the iliotibial band or gluteus maximus snapping over the greater trochanter [33,35,36]. The internal type is caused by the iliopsoas snapping over the iliopectineal eminence, the femoral head, or the lesser trochanter [33,35,36]. The intra-articular type can be caused by loose bodies, osteochondral fractures, labral tears, or synovial chondromatosis [33,35,36].

This disorder presents with insidious-onset hip snapping, with or without associated pain. Most patients can voluntarily reproduce the snapping and it is frequently palpable to the examiner. In a study of elite ballet dancers [35], *grand battement à la seconde* (straight-leg high kick to the side) produced symptoms in 41.8%, *grand plié* (deep squat with the hips externally rotated) in 25.3%, and *developpe à la seconde* (bent-leg kick developing into straight-leg kick to the side) in 22.8%. During physical examination, labral hip maneuver (alternating hip flexion and extension while lying on side) can reproduce external-type symptoms. FABERs maneuver may help elicit internal-type symptoms.

Ultrasound imaging is positive in 60% of tendonous cases [35]. "Psoas-gram," injection of contrast along the psoas tendon, can allow fluoroscopic visualization of the snapping tendon, but this is less often used. Magnetic resonance arthrogram is the imaging study of choice to evaluate intra-articular pathology. Treatment depends on the type of pathology associated with the snapping. All can benefit from nonsteroidal anti-inflammatory medication for pain management. For external type, stretching and active release therapy for the iliotibial band and gluteus maximus are the first line of treatment [36]. If indicated, steroid injection can be used to treat associated trochanteric bursitis. Stretching of the iliopsoas is the treatment of choice for internal snapping hip [35]. Surgical lengthening of the iliotibial band or iliopsoas may be used in very resistant, severe cases. The intra-articular type is treated surgically.

Sports hernias and groin disruptions

Sports hernias and groin disruptions are caused by posterior abdominal wall insufficiency and abnormalities. The literature often combines these two diagnoses or uses the terms interchangeably without precise definitions. Posterior inguinal wall weakening is most associated with the sports hernias, while groin disruptions appear to have a wider variety of causes, including tears or dehiscence of the conjoined tendon or inguinal ligament or tears of the external oblique aponeurosis [17,37]. Because no full-thickness wall lesions are involved, there is no true or palpable hernia.

Patients report insidious-onset exertional groin pain that may radiate into the anterior thigh, inguinal region, rectum, perineum, or scrotum. Valsalva maneuver may exacerbate pain in sports hernias, but is less common in groin disruption [17]. Tenderness with deep palpation to the inguinal region or low abdominal wall may or may not be present. Pain is frequently elicited with resisted hip flexion, adduction, or with half sit-ups [17] and supine pelvic lifts ("reverse crunch" targeting the lower abdomen/transversus abdominus).

Radiographs, MRI, CT scan, and bone scan can be helpful in ruling out other diagnoses, but most often do not show any abnormality in sports hernia or groin disruption. Initial conservative treatment with rest from sport followed by stretching and strengthening the lower abdomen and groin muscles is warranted. Many patients may continue to have symptoms despite rest and therapeutic exercise. Surgical exploration and repair are often required and are successful in improving symptoms in 90% to 95% of cases where lesions are found [38]. There are no significant potential complications other than persistent pain-related functional or athletic limitations.

Summary

Injuries relating to the lower extremity are quite varied, depending upon the age of the athlete, the sport, and the mechanism of injury. It is important for the sports medicine physician to evaluate the pediatric/adolescent athlete for any bony injuries, given the potential for subsequent surgery. Fortunately, injuries relating to muscle, ligaments, or tendons resolve with appropriate nonoperative treatment. With proper diagnosis and treatment, the athlete can return to sports quickly and, it is hoped, not experience future injuries.

References

[1] Waters PM, Millis MB. Hip and pelvic injuries in the young athlete. Clin Sports Med 1988;7: 513–26.

[2] Lee MC, Eberson CP. Growth and development of the child's hip. Orthop Clin N Am 2006;37(2):119–32.

[3] Weinstein SL, Mubarak SJ, Wnger DR. Developmental hip dysplasia and dislocation. Part I. Instr Course Lect 2004;53:523–30.

[4] Anderson SJ. Lower extremity injuries in youth sports. Pediatr Clin North Am 2002;49(3): 627–41.

[5] Millis MB, Kocher MS. Hip, pelvis, femur: pediatric aspects. In: Koval KJ, editor. Orthopaedic knowledge update 7. Chicago: American Academy of Orthopaedic Surgeons; 2002. p. 387–94.

[6] Kocher MS, Tucker R. Pediatric athlete hip disorders. Clin Sports Med 2006;25(2):241–53.

[7] Mehlman CT, Hubbard GW, Crawford AH, et al. Traumatic hip dislocation in children: long-term followup of 42 patients. Clin Orthop Relat Res 2000;376:68–79.

[8] Klenerman L. ABC of sports medicine: musculoskeletal injuries in child athletes. BMJ 1994; 308:1556–9.

[9] Quick TJ, Eastwood DM, Rodriguez-Merchan EC, et al. Pediatric fractures and dislocations of the hip and pelvis. Clin Orthop Relat Res 2005;432:87–96.

[10] Herring JA, Neustadt JB, Williams JJ, et al. The lateral pillar classification of Legg-Calvé-Perthes disease. J Pediatr Orthop 1992;12:143–50.

[11] Herring JA, Kim HT, Browne R. Legg-Calvé-Perthes disease. Part 1: classification of radiographs with use of the modified lateral pillar and Stulberg classifications. J Bone Joint Surg Am 2004;86(10):2103–20.

[12] Herring JA, Kim HT, Browne R. Legg-Calvé-Perthes disease. Part II: prospective multicenter study of the effect of treatment on outcome. J Bone Joint Surg Am 2004;86(10): 2121–34.

[13] Eckberg O, Persson NH, Abramson PA, et al. Longstanding groin pain in athletes. A multidisciplinary approach. Sports Med 1988;6:56–61.

[14] Rodrigeuz C, Miguel A, Lima H, et al. Osteitis pubis syndrome in a professional athlete: a case report. J Athl Train 2001;36:437–40.

[15] Haider NR, Syed RA, Dermandy D. Osteitis pubis—an important pain generator in women with lower pelvic or abdominal pain: a case report and literature review. Pain Physician 2005; 8(1):145–7.

[16] Fricker PA. Osteitis pubis. Sports Medicine and Arthroscopy Review 1997;5:305–12.

[17] Morelli V, Smith V. Groin injuries in athletes. Am Fam Physician 2001;64(8):1405–14.

[18] Karlsson J, Jerre R. The use of radiography, magnetic resonance, and ultrasound in the diagnosis of hip, pelvis, and groin injuries. Sports Medicine and Arthroscopy Review 1997;5:268–73.

[19] Hart E, Grottkau B, Albright M. Slipped capital femoral epiphysis: don't miss this pediatric hip disorder. Nurse Pract 2007;32(3):14–21.

[20] Lehman CL, Arons RR, Loder RT, et al. The epidemiology of slipped capital femoral epiphysis: an update. J Pediatr Orthop 2006;26(3):286–90.

[21] Loder RT, Aronson DD, Greenfield ML. The epidemiology of bilateral slipped capital femoral epiphysis. A study of children in Michigan. J Bone Joint Surg Am 1993;75:1141–7.

[22] Kehl DK. Slipped capital femoral epiphysis. In: Morrissy RT, Weinstein SL, editors. Lovell and Winter's pediatric orthopaedics. 5th edition. Philadelphia: Lippincott Williams and Wilkins; 2001. p. 999–1033.

[23] Umans H, Liebling MS, Moy L, et al. Slipped capital femoral epiphysis: a physical lesion diagnosed by MRI with radiographic and CT correlation. Skeletal Radiol 1998;27:139–44.

[24] Lubicky JP. Chondrolysis and avascular necrosis: complications of slipped capital femoral epiphysis. J Pediatr Orthop 1996;5:162–7.

[25] Belkin SC. Stress fractures in athletics. Orthop Clin North Am 1980;11(4):735–41.

[26] Tountas AA, Waddell JP. Stress fractures of the femoral neck. A report of seven cases. Clin Orthop Relat Res 1986;(210):160–5.

[27] Lin JT, Lane JM. Sacral stress fractures. J Womens Health 2003;12(9):879–88.

[28] Micheli LJ, Curtic C. Stress fractures in the spine and sacrum. Clin Sports Med 2006;25(1): 75–88.

[29] Blazina ME. The "hip-pointer," a term used to describe a specific kind of athletic injury. Calif Med 1967;106(6):450.

[30] Hoelmich P. Adductor related groin pain in athletes. Sports Medicine and Arthroscopy Review 1997;5:285–91.

[31] Renstrom P, Peterson L. Groin injuries in athletes. Br J Sports Med 1980;14:30–6.

[32] Lynch SA, Renstrom PA. Groin injuries in sport: treatment strategies. Sports Med 1999;28: 137–44.

[33] Dobbs MB, Gordon JE, Luhmann SJ, et al. Surgical correction of the snapping iliopsoas tendon in adolescents. J Bone Joint Surg Am 2002;84-A(3):420–4.

[34] Beals R. Painful snapping hip in young adults. West J Med 1993;159(4):481–2.

[35] Winston P, Awan R, Cassidy JD, et al. Clinical examination and ultrasound of self-reported snapping hip syndrome in elite ballet dancers. Am J Sports Med 2007;35(1):118–26.

[36] Idjadi J, Meslin R. Symptomatic snapping hip. Available at: www.physsportsmed.com. 2004;32(1):25–31. Accessed February 12, 2008.

[37] Gilmore J. Groin pain in the soccer athlete: fact, fiction, and treatment. Clin Sports Med 1998;17:787–93.

[38] Hackney RG. The sports hernia: a cause of chronic groin pain. Br J Sports Med 1993;27: 58–62.

PHYSICAL MEDICINE
AND REHABILITATION
CLINICS OF
NORTH AMERICA

ELSEVIER
SAUNDERS

Phys Med Rehabil Clin N Am
19 (2008) 319–345

Acute Knee Injuries in Skeletally Immature Athletes

Hua Ming Siow, MBChB, MMed, FRCSEd[a,b],
Danielle B. Cameron, BA[a],
Theodore J. Ganley, MD[a,c],*

[a]Department of Orthopaedic Surgery, Children's Hospital of Philadelphia, 2nd Floor,
Wood Center, 34th St. & Civic Center Blvd., Philadelphia, PA 19104, USA
[b]Department of Orthopaedic Surgery, KK Women's and Children's Hospital,
100 Bukit Timah Road, Singapore 229899
[c]The University of Pennsylvania School of Medicine, 2nd Floor, Wood Center,
34th St. & Civic Center Blvd., Philadelphia, PA 19104, USA

The knee is the body part most commonly injured as a consequence of collisions, falls, and overuse occurring from childhood sports [1]. The knee is also the site most prone to chronic and permanent disability [2]. The number of sports-related injuries is increasing because of active participation of children in competitive sports. Sports-related injuries account for one fourth of all injuries in children [3]. Approximately 30 million children are involved in organized sports, and up to a third of these children sustain an injury that requires medical attention [4]. Certain sports have increased potential for knee injuries, such as soccer, football, basketball, cycling, and Alpine sports [5,6].

Children differ from adults in many areas, such as increased rate and ability of healing, higher strength of ligaments compared with growth plates, and continued growth. Growth around the knee can be affected if the growth plates are involved in injuries. The distal femoral physis is the most active growth plate in the body and contributes approximately 1 cm of growth per year, which provides 70% of the growth of the femur and 37% of the growth of the lower limb. The proximal tibial physis contributes approximately 0.7 cm of growth per year and contributes 55% of the growth of the tibia and 25% of

* Corresponding author. Department of Orthopaedic Surgery, Children's Hospital of Philadelphia, 2nd Floor, Wood Center, 34th St. & Civic Center Blvd., Philadelphia, PA 19104.
 E-mail address: ganley@email.chop.edu (T.J. Ganley).

1047-9651/08/$ - see front matter. Published by Elsevier Inc.
doi:10.1016/j.pmr.2007.11.005

the growth of the lower limb [7–10]. Injuries to these active growth plates may result in significant limb length discrepancies or angular deformities.

Children often have inadequately developed motor skills and coordination. They may have intrinsic factors that predispose to injury, such as inadequate strength, flexibility, and endurance for their chosen sport. They also may have abnormal morphology or biomechanics. Extrinsic factors, such as poor training techniques and conditioning, poor supervision and coaching, lack of or improper use of safety equipment, excessive loading of the knee, and physical or psychologic stress, also contribute to injury.

History

The history initially should be directed toward the type of sport played, the equipment or footwear being worn, the playing surface, any history of direct trauma, and any history of previous injury. The magnitude and direction of force involved in the injury also should be assessed. Patients should be asked whether there was a pop or snap at the time of injury, whether there was a fall, and if it was possible to get up unassisted. They should be questioned about whether they were able to continue playing and for how long. Also questioned is the presence of swelling and the rapidity with which it occurred, which may differentiate a cruciate ligament injury, dislocation, or fracture from a meniscal injury or ligament sprain. Patients are asked whether there was any displacement of the patella and whether it reduced spontaneously. The onset of pain, and type, severity, and radiation of pain should be determined, as should any aggravating or relieving factors. Any history of crepitus, locking, or giving way of the knee after the injury is elicited, as is the medical treatment received and its effectiveness.

Physical examination

The neurovascular status of the lower limbs should be documented, followed by inspection of the leg at rest. It is assessed for the presence of intra-articular effusion, extra-articular swelling, ecchymosis, deformity, or quadriceps wasting. The coronal alignment of the knees and leg lengths should be determined. Children are asked where their pain is located, and palpation of that area is reserved for last so as not to upset children unnecessarily. Palpation should include the joint lines, physes of the distal femur and proximal tibia, femoral condyles, tibial plateau, pes anserinus, medial and lateral collateral ligaments (LCLs), proximal end of the fibula, tibial tuberosity, patella tendon, superior and inferior poles of the patella, patellar retinaculum, and quadriceps. Passive translation of the patella medially and laterally and apprehension testing should be performed.

Passive and active range of motion of the knee and patellar tracking are assessed, followed by stress testing of the anterior and posterior cruciate ligaments and medial and lateral collateral ligaments and provocative testing of the menisci. The presence of crepitus is noted if present. It is important to remember that ligaments are stronger than the bones or physes in children and that an apparent ligamentous instability may actually may be a physeal injury or fracture. It is also helpful to compare the stability of ligaments with those of the normal knee to avoid confusion in ligamentously lax individuals.

Range of motion of the hip should be assessed with minimal motion of the knee to avoid confusing the hip examination. Hip disorders such as slipped capital femoral epiphysis and Legg-Calvé-Perthes disease may refer pain to the knee. Ligamentous hypermobility also should be assessed. Gait examination should be performed if possible; however, the presence of acute injury and pain usually results in an antalgic gait, provided that the patient is able to walk unaided.

Investigations

Anteroposterior and lateral radiographs are routinely obtained. The Merchant or skyline views to visualize the patellofemoral articulation and the anteroposterior notch view to visualize the posterior aspect of the femoral condyles may be helpful. Oblique radiographs may help to reveal subtle fractures. MRI or CT is useful in further evaluation of bones and soft tissue, which is especially true when the injury is not apparent on plain radiographs and there is a preceding traumatic event, effusion, or swelling together with a refusal to weight bear on the leg [11].

The use of radiographs may be decreased by 31% with the use of the Ottawa Knee Rules, which have a sensitivity of 100% and specificity of 43% for detecting a fracture [12]. Although MRI of the knee has been shown to have a sensitivity of 92% to 100% and a specificity of 87% to 100% [13], Kocabey and colleagues [14] have shown that there was no difference between MRI and a well-trained orthopedic surgeon in terms of ability to diagnose intra-articular soft tissue knee injuries.

Fractures

Distal femoral physeal fractures

These fractures are relatively uncommon, accounting for 7% of physeal injuries of the lower extremities [15,16]. The distal femoral physis has a complex shape with four depressions, into which four matching processes of the distal femoral metaphysis fit. This shape provides increased resistance to shear but also results in an increased risk of focal damage to the physis if injury occurs because of the decreased odds of a "clean" cleavage plane across the physis [17]. Juvenile injuries occur mostly after a high-velocity trauma, such as a motor vehicle accident (44% of injuries), whereas adolescent injuries occur mainly in relatively low-energy activities, such as sports

(25% of injuries) [9,18–20]. Hyperextension is the most common mechanism of injury. Individuals who play sports that involve jumping, such as high jump, hurdles, and basketball, have a higher incidence of this injury [21].

The commonly used classification for physeal injuries is that of Salter and Harris (Fig. 1) [22]. In type I fractures, there is separation through the physis with no metaphyseal or epiphyseal involvement. Type II fractures are the most common physeal injuries in this area and form 54% of all injuries [18–20]. The fracture line traverses the physis before exiting obliquely through the metaphysis. The metaphyseal fragment (Thurston-Holland fragment) is often opposite the direction of force, and the physis attached to it is least susceptible to growth arrest because the physis is not disrupted. Type III fractures consist of a fracture through the physis that exits through the epiphysis into the joint (Fig. 2 A–D). Type IV fractures consist of a fracture line that crosses the metaphysis, physis, and epiphysis into the joint. Type V fractures are crush injuries to the physeal cartilage. They are rare and difficult to diagnose initially, often presenting 6 to 12 months later with limb shortening or angular deformity. Comparison radiographs of the normal contralateral physis may distinguish narrowing of the injured physis.

Undisplaced fractures are treated with immobilization in an above-knee cast or hip spica for 4 to 6 weeks. Serial weekly radiographs for 3 weeks help to exclude secondary displacement. Gentle closed reduction is attempted for displaced type I and II fractures because excessive manipulation can damage the growth plate. The common rule is 90% traction and 10% manipulation. Fractures with greater displacement, especially hyperextension injuries, are associated with an increased risk of displacement, thus percutaneous fixation is recommended [23]. Large thigh girths make cast immobilization more difficult and may indicate fixation to maintain reduction [17]. Open reduction may be necessary if closed reduction is unsuccessful (Fig. 3 A, B).

Types I and II fractures can be fixed with one or two smooth pins from the epiphysis to the metaphysis. These pins are bent and left under the skin, with removal after fracture healing. If the Thurston-Holland fragment is large enough, type II fractures can be fixed with percutaneous screws across

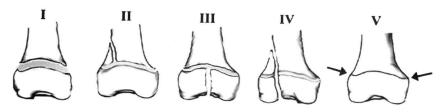

Fig. 1. Salter-Harris fracture classification. (*From* Flynn JM, Skaggs D, Sponseller PD, et al. The operative management of pediatric fractures of the lower extremity. J Bone Joint Surg Am 2002;84(12):2292; with permission.)

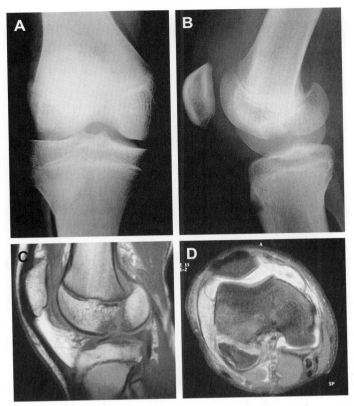

Fig. 2. (*A*) Anteroposterior radiograph. Displaced distal femoral physeal fracture, Salter-Harris type III. (*B*) Lateral radiograph, (*C*) T1-weighted MRI sagittal view, (*D*) T2-weighted MRI, axial view.

the fragment and into the metaphyseal area. Types III and IV fractures are fixed with intra-epiphyseal screws [24] and usually require open reduction to anatomically reduce to joint line. Failure to achieve anatomic reduction may result in the formation of an osseous bar, which can result in limb length discrepancy and angular deformity [9].

These injuries are frequently complicated by limb length discrepancy, angular deformity, stiffness of the knee, or neurovascular compromise. Riseborough and colleagues [20] found that younger children aged 2 to 11 with displaced fractures more than half the diameter of the femoral shaft were more likely to have subsequent growth problems. Angular deformity occurs in 24% of patients and limb length discrepancy in 32% [9]. Detection of these injuries requires at least 6 to 12 months of follow-up. Physeal injuries have even been noted in nonphyseal fractures of the lower limb, causing angular deformity that was noted on average 22 months after the injury [25]. MRI is used to determine if physeal osseous bars are present. Resection

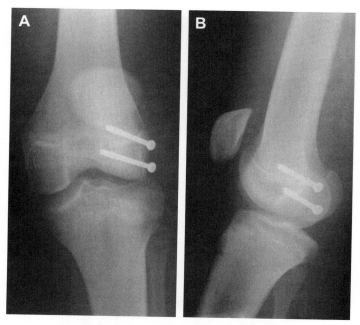

Fig. 3. (*A*) Postoperative radiographs, anteroposterior view, of distal femoral Salter-Harris type III physeal fracture with fixation with two cannulated screws. (*B*) Postoperative radiographs, lateral view, of distal femoral Salter-Harris type III physeal fracture.

is indicated if less than 50% of the physis is involved and there are more than 2 years of growth remaining (Fig. 4) [26]. Angular deformity is corrected by completion epiphysiodesis or osteotomy. Limb length discrepancy of less than 5 cm can be treated with contralateral epiphysiodesis, whereas discrepancy of more than 5 cm can be treated with limb lengthening or contralateral shortening procedures.

Neurovascular injuries are rare and occur in 2% of fractures [9]. Hyperextension injuries result in anterior displacement of the femoral physis and may injure the closely attached popliteal artery, whereas varus angulation may injure the peroneal nerve. Vascular injuries require immediate reduction and fixation of the fracture and on-table angiogram and vascular repair as necessary.

Proximal tibial physeal fractures

These fractures are rare and account for 3% of physeal injuries of the lower extremities [15,16]. Their incidence is half that of distal femoral physeal injuries, which is theorized to be caused by the collateral ligament and tendon insertions being located mainly in the metaphysis rather than the epiphysis, as compared with the distal femoral physis [27]. The mechanism

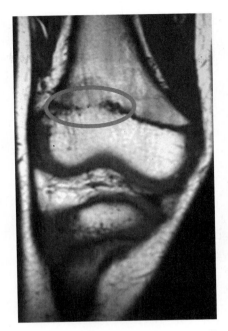

Fig. 4. Growth arrest of lateral distal femoral physis on T1-weighted MRI.

of injury is usually a hyperextension force that results in an apex posterior angulation of the metaphysis. This force can injure the popliteal artery, which is tethered by the anterior tibial artery, as it perforates the interosseous membrane. The fracture subsequently can reduce to an innocuous position on radiographs [28], so care must be taken to assess the neurovascular status of the limb.

The most common fractures are Salter-Harris type II (43%), followed by type III (22%), type IV (17%), type I (15%), and type V (2%) [28–30]. Most type I and II fractures can be treated with closed reduction and immobilization (Fig. 5 A–C). Types III and IV fractures can be treated with closed reduction and percutaneous pinning or screw fixation. Open reduction is indicated if anatomic reduction cannot be achieved, and for type II fractures this is rarely caused by pes anserinus interpositioned in the fracture site [31,32].

The most common complications are angular deformity (28%) and limb length discrepancy (19%), which mainly occur after open lawnmower injuries that damage the perichondral ring of the proximal tibial physis [28,30]. Vascular injury occurs in 5% to 7% of cases [28,30] and necessitates immediate reduction and fixation of the fracture and angiography and revascularization as appropriate. More uncommonly, anterior compartment syndrome, peroneal nerve palsy, and ligamentous and meniscal injuries can occur.

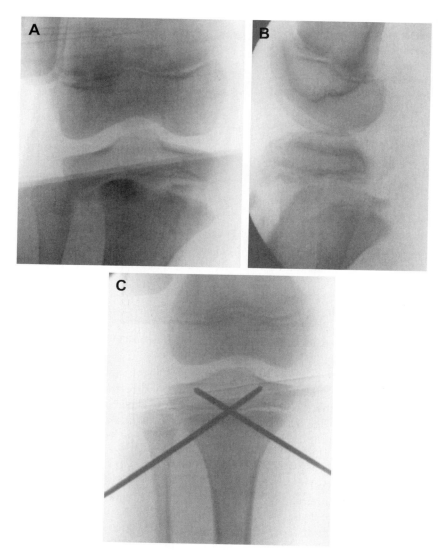

Fig. 5. (*A*) Anteroposterior radiograph of displaced proximal tibial Salter-Harris type II physeal fracture. (*B*) Lateral radiograph of displaced proximal tibial Salter-Harris type II physeal fracture. (*C*) After fixation with two crossed smooth pins.

Tibial tuberosity fractures

These fractures are Salter-Harris type III avulsion fractures of the proximal tibial physis [22] and account for 14% to 15% of proximal tibial fractures [28,30]. Watson-Jones [33] believed they were caused by either a violent contraction of the quadriceps muscle or sudden passive flexion of the knee against a contracted quadriceps muscle. Böhler [34] described them as being the result of "jumps with a bad landing." Ninety percent are sports related, and they occur at an average age of 15 [31,35–38]. They should be differentiated from Osgood-Schlatter's disease, which is a stress reaction of the anterior ossicle of the tuberosity with no involvement of the physis. The presence of acute symptoms for a tibial tuberosity fracture should help distinguish it from Osgood-Schlatter's disease. Ogden and colleagues [37] suggested that Osgood-Schlatter's disease predisposed to acute avulsion of the tibial tuberosity and found this association in 56% of his patients. Other authors have noted it in only 10% of patients, however [35,36,39].

Ogden and colleagues [37] modified the classification by Watson-Jones [33] to place more emphasis on intra-articular extension of the fracture and comminution of the tuberosity. Type I fractures involve a small avulsed fragment of the tuberosity, which is displaced upward. Type IA fractures are incompletely separated from the metaphysis, whereas type IB fractures are completely separated. Type II fractures involve the entire tibial tuberosity without extension of the fracture line into the proximal tibial epiphysis. Type IIA fractures are not comminuted, whereas IIB fractures are comminuted. Type III fractures extend proximally into the anterior tibial epiphysis and involve the articular surface. Type IIIA fractures are not comminuted, whereas IIIB fractures are comminuted.

Patients with type I fractures are usually able to actively extend their knee except against resistance, whereas patients with type II and III fractures are usually unable to extend the knee. Patella alta may be present depending on the amount of displacement of the tuberosity. Lateral radiographs in slight internal rotation afford the best view of the fracture. Undisplaced type I fractures are treated with a cast in extension for 6 weeks. Small type I avulsed fragments are treated by attaching tendon-holding sutures in the patella tendon and anchoring them to a screw in the proximal tibia. Larger fragments are fixed directly to the metaphysis with screws for older adolescents or K-wires and periosteal sutures for children, followed by casting at 30° for 4 to 6 weeks (Fig. 6 A–D). Intra-articular fractures require inspection of the joint surface for anatomic reduction and to visualize any associated meniscal tears, detachment, or interfragmentary entrapment [40]. Progressive rehabilitation of the quadriceps continues until normal strength is achieved with full range of motion of the knee. Sports activities are allowed 3 to 5 months after the injury [36,37].

Complications are rare. Genu recurvatum may develop in the rare tuberosity fracture before the age of 11 (Fig. 7) [9,41,42]. Damage to the anterior tibial recurrent artery in the region of the tibial tuberosity has been reported to cause compartment syndrome [43,44], and patients should be monitored closely for this condition postoperatively.

Tibial eminence fractures

The anterior tibial eminence, or spine, is the site of insertion for the anterior cruciate ligament (ACL). Before ossification of the proximal physis

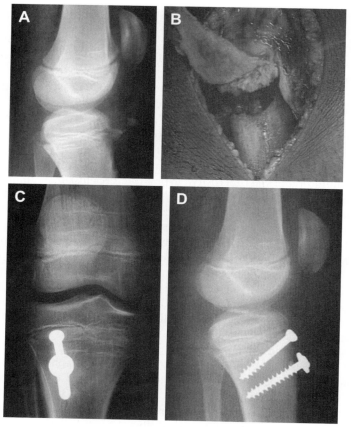

Fig. 6. (*A*) Preoperative lateral radiograph of tibial tuberosity fracture. (*B*) Intraoperative view during open reduction of tibial tuberosity fracture. (*C*) Anteroposterior radiograph of tibial tuberosity fracture after fixation with two cancellous screws. (*D*) Lateral radiograph of tibial tuberosity fracture after fixation with two cancellous screws.

is complete, the insertion consists of a chondroepiphysis, which is weaker than the ACL. Traumatic forces, which in a mature individual would cause an ACL tear, usually result in a tibial eminence fracture in a child. These injuries account for 2% of knee injuries in children [45,46] and typically occur between the ages of 8 and 14. They are commonly associated with falls from bicycles that result in forceful hyperextension of the knee or a direct blow on the distal end of the femur with the knee flexed [47–50]. Decreased intercondylar notch width has been associated with decreased ACL size and increased risk of ACL rupture [51].

Meyers and McKeever [49] classified these fractures according to the amount of displacement and the fracture pattern. Type I fractures are minimally displaced (Fig. 8). Type II fractures have a posterior hinge with an

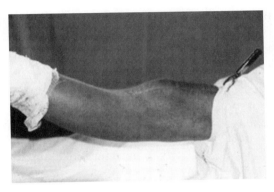

Fig. 7. Genu recurvatum.

elevated anterior portion. Type III fractures are completely displaced fragments and may be rotated. Zaricznyj [52] has added a type IV, which are
comminuted fractures of the tibial eminence.

Radiographs often underestimate the size of the largely cartilaginous fragment, and MRI may be useful for further assessment [40]. Types I and II
fractures, which can be reduced by closed means, are treated with cast immobilization in 10° of flexion for 6 weeks, followed by rehabilitation. Failure of
closed reduction is usually caused by interposed medial or lateral meniscus
or the intermeniscal ligament. Irreducible types II and III fractures require
open or arthroscopic reduction and fixation. Fixation may consist of

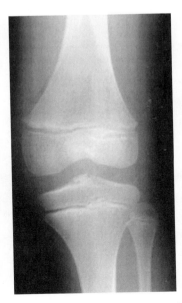

Fig. 8. Minimally displaced tibial eminence fractures.

K-wire, suture, or screw fixation, either transphyseal or intraepiphyseal. Transphyseal wires or screws require operative removal after fracture union.

Complications include arthrofibrosis, residual laxity and instability, extension loss, extension block from malunion, nonunion, and prominence or irritation of fixation devices [53]. Residual anterior laxity has been reported in up to 64% of patients at 4 years follow-up, regardless of treatment method [50]. Wiley and colleagues [50] did not report any long-term functional instability, whereas Grönkvist and colleagues [48] found functional instability in 38% of their patients and noted that children younger than age 10 were much less likely to have functional instability.

Patellar fractures

Patellar fractures make up less than 5% of all knee injuries [54,55] and are uncommon because of the large ratio of cartilage to bone, increased mobility, and tissue resilience [9]. These fractures result from direct trauma or avulsion forces across the patella. Most fractures are caused by motor vehicle accidents, and only 17% are related to sports [55,56]. Direct trauma in older adolescents usually results in a transverse fracture of the patella. Sleeve fractures occur when an extensive sleeve of cartilage is avulsed off the main body of the patella along with a bony fragment from the distal pole (Fig. 9) [57]. These fractures can be missed on radiographs because of the radiolucent sleeve of cartilage and small bony fragments.

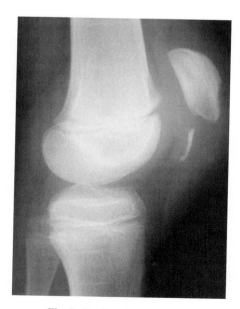

Fig. 9. Patellar sleeve fracture.

The knee is swollen, usually with an extension lag, palpable gap in the extensor mechanism, and patella alta. Minimally displaced fractures, which allow active extension, can be treated with a long leg cast for 4 to 6 weeks. Displaced fractures or disruption of the extensor mechanism requires open reduction and internal fixation with the tension band technique, a circumferential wire loop, or interfragmentary screws. The patella retinaculum is repaired at the same time (Fig. 10).

Outcomes are generally good. Results are poor with more displaced and comminuted fractures [56]. Inadequate reduction or fixation can result in patella alta, extensor lag, and quadriceps muscle atrophy [9].

Patellar dislocation

The incidence of acute patellar dislocation in children between ages 9 and 15 has been reported as 1 in 1000 per year [58]. The typical mechanism is an indirect twisting injury, with the femur internally rotating over a planted foot and valgus knee. This is a similar mechanism of injury for ACL tears, which should be excluded during the assessment of this injury. Other mechanisms include a direct trauma to the lateral aspect of the knee or medial edge of the patella. Predisposing factors include patella alta, abnormal patellar morphology, lateral patellar displacement, trochlear dysplasia, increased Q angle, genu valgum, vastus medialis hypoplasia, ligament hyperlaxity, external tibia torsion, subtalar joint pronation, and increased femoral anteversion [59]. The Q angle is defined as the angle formed at the center of the

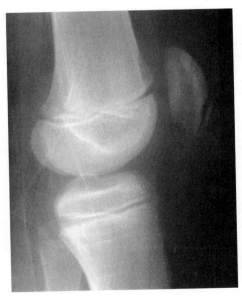

Fig. 10. Patellar sleeve fracture suture repair. See Fig. 11.

patella by the line of pull of the quadriceps tendon and that of the patellar tendon. This angle is normally 15° or less, and a larger angle would indicate an increased tendency for lateral subluxation of the patella.

The patella is typically dislocated laterally, and spontaneous reduction usually occurs with the knee in extension. Occasionally, the patient presents with a painful flexed knee and persistent dislocation. Immediate reduction is performed with the patient being as relaxed as possible and bringing the knee to full extension, with gentle medializing pressure on the dislocated patella if necessary. Examination reveals medial retinacular tenderness and a positive apprehension test. Palpation of the patella and femoral articular surfaces may reveal tenderness over chondral or osteochondral injuries.

Treatment of first-time patellar dislocations is by immobilization of the knee in extension for 3 weeks. A lateral compression pad also can be added [60]. Quadriceps isometrics, straight leg raises, and single plane motion exercises begin early. Relative indications for early surgical treatment include the presence of an osteochondral fracture, substantial disruption of the medial patellar stabilizers, laterally subluxated patella with normal patellar alignment in the contralateral knee, recurrent dislocation, and lack of improvement with appropriate rehabilitation [59]. Rorabeck and Bobechko [61] described three patterns of fracture for osteochondral fractures associated with patellar dislocations: inferomedial fracture of the patella, fracture of the lateral femoral condyle, and a combination of the two (Fig. 11). They estimated that it occurred in 5% of patellar dislocations, but Nietosvaara and colleagues [58] reported an incidence of 39%, whereas Stanitski and colleagues [62] reported a 71% incidence of articular injury on arthroscopy. MRI is more effective than plain radiographs at visualizing fragments, which are largely cartilaginous, and helps to visualize injuries to the medial patellar stabilizers and articular surfaces (Fig. 12 A–C) [63,64]. The presence of an osteochondral fracture is an indication for surgery, which may range from arthroscopic excision of small fragments from non–weight-bearing surfaces to fixation of larger fragments from weight-bearing surfaces using Herbert screws or biodegradable

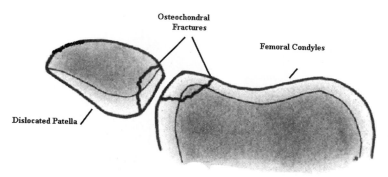

Fig. 11. Common locations for osteochondral fractures of femoral condyle and patella with dislocation of patella.

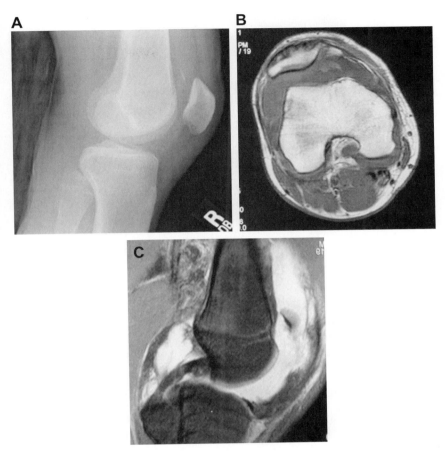

Fig. 12. (*A*) Lateral radiograph of osteochondral fracture of the patella. (*B*) Axial view of T1-weighted MRI. (*C*) Sagittal view of T2-weighted MRI.

pins. If fixation is used, weight bearing should be avoided until radiographic healing occurs. Chondral injuries can be treated with débridement, microfracture, or drilling for smaller defects. Larger defects may require the use of resurfacing techniques, such as osteochondral autograft or autologous chondrocyte implantation.

The medial patellofemoral ligament (MPFL) has been shown to provide 50% to 60% of the total restraining force to patellar displacement [65–68]. Disruption of this ligament and medial patellar retinaculum, as visualized on MRI, occurs in 76% to 81% of patellar dislocations (Fig. 13) [64,69]. Surgical studies have identified 94% to 100% injury to the medial patellofemoral ligament with patellar dislocations [70–72]. It is becoming more accepted to repair or reconstruct the medial patellofemoral ligament either acutely or for recurrent patellar dislocations [73,74].

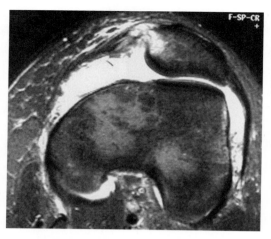

Fig. 13. T2-weighted MRI axial view of medial patellofemoral ligament/medial retinacular disruption.

The rate of redislocation for conservatively treated first-time patellar dislocations is approximately 29% compared with 17% for operatively treated patients [59]. Other long-term complications include patellar instability, pain, decreased level of sporting activity, and patellofemoral arthritis.

Anterior cruciate ligament injuries

These injuries have been reported to occur in 16 per 1000 high school athletes annually [75]. Female athletes who participate in basketball and soccer have a higher incidence of ACL ruptures. The mechanism of injury is usually hyperextension, sudden deceleration, or a valgus and rotatory force with a planted foot. There may be a "pop" sensation at the time of injury, and a large effusion often develops within a few hours. Athletes are unable to continue play and are unable to bear weight on the injured limb. Acute assessment is difficult because of hemarthrosis and pain. The Lachman test is the most sensitive for assessing ACL injury. Anterior drawer and pivot shift tests are also useful, if more difficult to perform acutely. Approximately 22% to 65% of ACL tears have been judged to be partial on arthroscopy [76–78]. Partial tears that involve more than 50% of the ACL lead to symptoms of instability and should be managed as full-thickness tears. Associated medial collateral ligament (MCL) and meniscal injuries occur frequently, so a thorough assessment is useful. ACL injuries can be confused with patellar dislocations and tibial eminence fractures, so these diagnoses should be borne in mind during the evaluation.

Standard radiographs of the knee are taken to assess for the presence of avulsion fractures, lateral capsular avulsions, and osteochondral fractures.

Wrist films are useful for assessing the bone age of the patient. MRI evaluation of ACL injuries in young patients correlated with arthroscopic findings has revealed a sensitivity of 95% and a specificity of 88% (Fig. 14). They also give information on meniscal and chondral injuries.

There is an inherent risk of iatrogenic physeal injury with surgical intervention near an open physis. The adoption of a management strategy for ACL injuries is related to the skeletal maturity of the individual and the potential for further growth. Tanner and Davies [79] noted that the adolescent growth spurt begins at an average of 10.5 years in girls and 12.5 years in boys, with peak velocity at 11.5 years in girls and 13.5 years in boys. Determination of skeletal maturity requires correlation of Tanner staging, assessment of bone age with the Greulich and Pyle [80] atlas, menarche in girls, family height, and cessation in changes in shoe size [81].

Nonoperative treatment for ACL injuries includes bracing of the knee, restoration of range of motion, strengthening the quadriceps and hamstrings, and activity modification. Most children have difficulty restricting their activity levels, which eventually results in progressive damage to the articular cartilage and menisci [77,82–87]. This damage usually leads to compromised knee function and chronic osteoarticular changes as they age [82].

Surgical intervention should be undertaken only after restoration of the range of motion. Acute repair of ACL tears has not met with great success, and most patients continue to have recurrent instability after operation [88,89]. The surgical options consist of physeal sparing, partial transphyseal, or complete transphyseal ACL reconstructions, which are usually intra-articular, although combined intra- and extra-articular

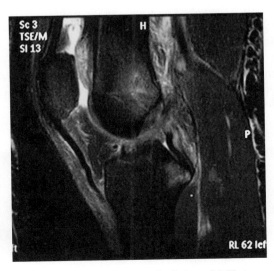

Fig. 14. T2-weighted MRI sagittal view of ACL tear.

reconstructions are popular if the physes are being avoided. Allograft may be used with good results [90], although traditionally hamstring grafts have been used. The iliotibial band also has been used in combined intra- and extra-articular reconstructions [91]. Advantages of autografts include no risk of disease transmission or immune reactions; disadvantages include increased operative time and graft donor site complications. Advantages of allograft include ready availability of graft sizes, lack of donor site complications, shorter operative time, possible decrease in postoperative pain, and easier rehabilitation. Disadvantages of allograft consist of the slight risk of disease transmission, the potential for an immune reaction, and concerns about prolonged shelf life affecting their structural properties.

If nonoperative treatment is unsuccessful or the child is determined to perform at a high level in sports, surgical reconstruction is an option for immature patients. An associated meniscal tear is also an indication for operation. An immature patient with Tanner stage of 0 or 1 may require a physeal-sparing reconstruction. Guzzanti and colleagues [92] used a physeal-sparing intra-articular technique, Anderson [93] used an intra-articular technique, and Kocher and colleagues [94] used a combined intra- and extra-articular reconstruction, all with good results. Patients who are Tanner stage 2 can undergo a partial transphyseal reconstruction whereby the tibial tunnel is transphyseal and the femoral fixation is physeal sparing; these procedures have been safe and effective [95–99]. Patients who are stage 3 and higher or with a bone age of 13 for girls and 14 for boys, may undergo complete transphyseal techniques with central tunnels 6 to 9 mm in diameter, which are filled with soft tissue graft [100,101]. Excessive tension is avoided [102]. This is similar to adult-type ACL reconstructions and is usually used in skeletally mature adolescents who have completed their growth spurt [85,87,90,103]. The same techniques recently have been used in skeletally immature patients with good results (Fig. 15 A, B) [82,104,105].

Complications are rare and include angular deformity, such as genu valgum, genu recurvatum from premature closure of the tibial tuberosity apophysis, limb length discrepancy, rupture of the graft, arthrofibrosis, and donor site complications [98,106,107]. Recommendations to avoid previously mentioned complications include avoidance of hardware or bone

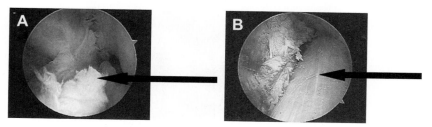

Fig. 15. (A) Arthroscopic view of ACL tear. (B) Arthroscopic view of reconstructed ACL.

crossing the physis, central location of tunnels, tunnels not exceeding 9 mm in diameter, tunnels that are completely filled with soft tissue graft, and avoidance of physeal injury in fixation and placement of grafts. A good postoperative rehabilitation program to restore knee motion, stability, and strength is crucial, with return to sports at 6 months provided athletes have full range of motion, good stability, and 80% of quadriceps and hamstring strength of the other leg.

Posterior cruciate ligament injuries

These injuries are rare in children, with only case reports in the literature. The mechanism of injury is a posteriorly directed force to the tibia with the knee flexed at 90° or by knee hyperextension. Patients may present with a decreased range of motion of the knee, inability to bear weight on the injured limb, or posterior joint line tenderness [108]. The posterior drawer test at 90° of knee flexion is usually positive. An unsuspected posterior cruciate ligament injury can result in a posterior sag that may produce a false-positive anterior drawer sign and cause confusion with an ACL injury.

Radiographs may show avulsion fractures of the origin or insertion of the posterior cruciate ligament, and an MRI helps to confirm the diagnosis. Avulsion fractures are treated by primary repair with screws or sutures. Midsubstance ruptures are treated conservatively with range-of-motion and muscle-strengthening exercises. Reconstruction at skeletal maturity is considered if there is persistent pain or instability.

Collateral ligament injuries

The MCL is more commonly injured than the LCL. MCL injuries occur from a valgus or external rotation force to the knee when the foot is planted, commonly while playing football or soccer. Physeal injuries tend to predominate in younger patients, whereas more skeletally mature adolescents tend to sustain MCL injuries. There is swelling and tenderness over the MCL. Laxity with valgus stress testing at 30° of knee flexion occurs with higher grade tears, whereas laxity with valgus stress at full knee extension indicates further damage to the posteromedial capsule and cruciate ligaments (Fig. 16).

Isolated MCL tears are treated conservatively [109]. Concurrent injuries to the menisci or ACL may necessitate surgical treatment, however. In concurrent MCL and ACL injuries, bracing of higher grade injuries for a month followed by ACL reconstruction has produced good results [110].

LCL injuries occur when a varus force is directed to the knee or in knee hyperextension, and external rotation may be involved. There is tenderness and swelling over the LCL. LCL injuries are frequently associated with other injuries, such as posterolateral corner, ACL, and posterior cruciate ligament injuries. Peroneal nerve injuries need to be excluded with combined LCL and posterolateral corner injuries [111]. Varus stress testing at 0° and 30° assesses

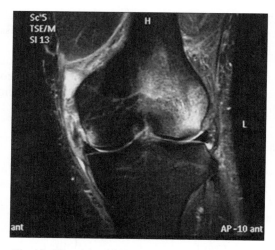

Fig. 16. T2-weighted MRI sagittal view of MCL tear.

the integrity of the LCL and posterolateral corner, and significant laxity may arise with concurrent ACL and posterior cruciate ligament injuries.

Isolated MCL and LCL injuries are treated in a similar fashion. The knee is initially immobilized, followed by early mobilization and strengthening exercises. Ice and nonsteroidal anti-inflammatory drugs are helpful during this phase. Hinged knee braces are used for 4 to 6 weeks. Return to sports is allowed when the patient is asymptomatic, has full range of motion and strength of the knee, and is able to perform sports-specific drills.

Meniscal injuries

Meniscal injuries in children younger than age 10 are rare unless they have a predisposing factor, such as a discoid meniscus. Clark and Ogden [112] have attributed this to the greater reparative potential of young children because of increased vascularity and cellularity, as compared with adolescents and adults. These injuries are seen more commonly in adolescent athletes and are frequently associated with ACL injuries, tibial eminence fractures, and chondral injuries [78,113,114]. Sports are the usual cause of injury as the result of a twisting mechanism or direct trauma that causes varus or valgus distortion of the knee. Athletes may present with pain, swelling, stiffness, instability, clicking, locking, or popping of the knee joint. Joint line tenderness may be the most consistent sign in children, whereas McMurray's test is less sensitive in children compared with adults. Stanitski [115] reported a sensitive test for medial meniscal injury whereby the knee is flexed at 30° to 40° and a varus and rotational stress is applied to the knee, resulting in medial joint line pain. The reverse applies for lateral meniscal tears.

Although MRI imaging for assessment of meniscal tears has improved recently—reaching 93% sensitivity and 95% specificity in a recent study [13]—clinical correlation has been shown to be more accurate than MRI alone [116]. The gold standard for diagnosis, as in all intra-articular pathology, is arthroscopy (Fig. 17 A–C).

The peripheral red-red zone of menisci is the most vascular and has the greatest potential for healing. The white-white zone is the most central and most avascular. The red-white zone is between these two zones and has intermediate vascularity. Most meniscal tears seen in children and adolescents are peripheral detachments of the meniscus, complete longitudinal tears, and bucket handle tears [117,118]. Tears in the red-red zone that are less than 1 cm long and have less than 3 mm of displacement can be treated without surgery. These knees are placed in a hinged knee brace with restricted flexion for 3 to 4 weeks. Arthroscopic repair is indicated for simple longitudinal peripheral tears in the red-red and red-white zones. Repairs can consist of inside-out, outside-in, and all-inside techniques using

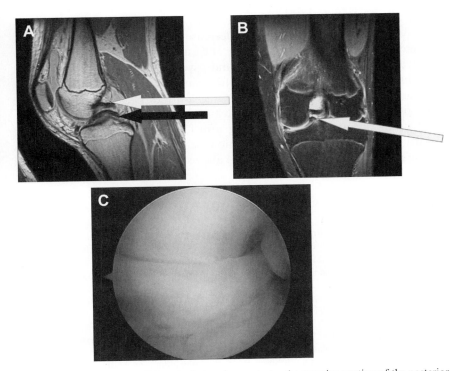

Fig. 17. (A) T1-weighted MRI sagittal view demonstrates the superior portion of the posterior cruciate ligament (*white arrow*) and a bucket handle medial meniscal tear (*black arrow*). (B) T2-weighted MRI coronal view of bucket handle tear and medial meniscal tear shows a portion of meniscus interposed within the intercondylar notch (*arrow*). (C) Arthroscopic view of bucket handle medial meniscal tear.

sutures or bioabsorbable fixation devices. Complex tears require débridement and contouring of the meniscus. Tears in the white-white zone are excised. Maximal preservation of stable meniscus is the aim of arthroscopic débridement. Postoperatively, the knee is immobilized in extension for 4 to 6 weeks with occasional range-of-motion exercises, limiting flexion to 60°. Full range of motion and weight bearing occurs progressively, with removal of the brace at 8 to 10 weeks.

Complications include neurovascular injury, infection, deep venous thrombosis, complex regional pain syndrome, intra-articular displacement of the fixation device, inadequate tensioning, and chondral injury [119–124].

Injury prevention

Hergenroeder [125] has outlined six potential strategies for reducing injuries in youth sports: (1) preseason physical examination, (2) medical coverage at sporting events, (3) proper coaching, (4) adequate hydration, (5) proper officiating, and (6) proper equipment and field/surface playing conditions. Training intensity should not be increased by more than 10% per week. Increased training intensity has been shown to relate to injury [126]. Proprioceptive training has been shown to decrease the risk of ACL injuries [127]. Athletes should be encouraged to have at least 2 days off per week from competitive sports to recover physically and psychologically. They also should abstain from any specific sport for 2 to 3 months a year [128]. Other issues correlated with injury include excessive pressure to perform well in sports, poor psychologic coping skills, and lack of social support [129].

It is important to educate young athletes, parents, and coaches with regard to ensuring proper rest, nutrition, safety, and training, which helps young athletes to prevent injuries and allows them to enjoy their participation in sporting activities.

References

[1] Backx FJ, Beijer HJ, Bol E, et al. Injuries in high-risk persons and high-risk sports: a longitudinal study of 1818 school children. Am J Sports Med 1991;19(2):124–30.

[2] Kujala UM, Taimela S, Antti-Poika I, et al. Acute injuries in soccer, ice hockey, volleyball, basketball, judo, and karate: analysis of national registry data. BMJ 1995;311(7018):1465–8.

[3] Ganley TJ, Pill SG, Flynn JM, et al. Pediatric sports medicine. Current Opinion in Orthopaedics 2001;12:457–61.

[4] Adirim TA, Cheng TL. Pediatric sports medicine. Pediatric sports medicine 2001;12:4–81.

[5] US Consumer Product Safety Commission National Electronic Injury Surveillance System (NEISS) database. Washington, DC: 2001.

[6] Deibert MC, Aronsson DD, Johnson RJ, et al. Skiing injuries in children, adolescents, and adults. J Bone Joint Surg Am 1998;80(1):25–32.

[7] Ogden JA. Skeletal injury in the child. 2nd edition. Philadelphia: Lea and Febiger; 1990.

[8] Shapiro F. Pediatric orthopaedic deformities: basic science, diagnosis, and treatment. San Diego (CA): Academic Press; 2001.

[9] Beaty JH, Kumar A. Fractures about the knee in children. J Bone Joint Surg Am 1994; 76(12):1870–80.

[10] Pritchett JW. Longitudinal growth and growth-plate activity in the lower extremity. Clin Orthop Relat Res 1992;(275):274–9.

[11] Naranja RJ Jr, Gregg JR, Dormans JP, et al. Pediatric fracture without radiographic abnormality: description and significance. Clin Orthop Relat Res 1997;(342):141–6.

[12] Bulloch B, Neto G, Plint A, et al. Validation of the Ottawa Knee Rule in children: a multi-center study. Ann Emerg Med 2003;42(1):48–55.

[13] Major NM, Beard LN Jr, Helms CA. Accuracy of MR imaging of the knee in adolescents. AJR Am J Roentgenol 2003;180(1):17–9.

[14] Kocabey Y, Tetik O, Isbell WM, et al. The value of clinical examination versus magnetic resonance imaging in the diagnosis of meniscal tears and anterior cruciate ligament rupture. Arthroscopy 2004;20(7):696–700.

[15] Mann DC, Rajmaira S. Distribution of physeal and nonphyseal fractures in 2,650 long-bone fractures in children aged 0-16 years. J Pediatr Orthop 1990;10(6):713–6.

[16] Peterson CA, Peterson HA. Analysis of the incidence of injuries to the epiphyseal growth plate. J Trauma 1972;12(4):275–81.

[17] Flynn JM, Skaggs DL, Sponseller PD, et al. The surgical management of pediatric fractures of the lower extremity. Instr Course Lect 2003;52:647–59.

[18] Czitrom AA, Salter RB, Willis RB. Fractures involving the distal epiphyseal plate of the femur. Int Orthop 1981;4(4):269–77.

[19] Lombardo SJ, Harvey JP Jr. Fractures of the distal femoral epiphyses: factors influencing prognosis. A review of thirty-four cases. J Bone Joint Surg Am 1977;59(6):742–51.

[20] Riseborough EJ, Barrett IR, Shapiro F. Growth disturbances following distal femoral physeal fracture-separations. J Bone Joint Surg Am 1983;65(7):885–93.

[21] Stephens DC, Louis E, Louis DS. Traumatic separation of the distal femoral epiphyseal cartilage plate. J Bone Joint Surg Am 1974;56(7):1383–90.

[22] Salter RB, Harris WR. Injuries involving the epiphyseal plate. J Bone Joint Surg Am 1963; 45(A):587–622.

[23] Thomson JD, Stricker SJ, Williams MM. Fractures of the distal femoral epiphyseal plate. J Pediatr Orthop 1995;15(4):474–8.

[24] Torg JS, Pavlov H, Morris VB. Salter-Harris type-III fracture of the medial femoral condyle occurring in the adolescent athlete. J Bone Joint Surg Am 1981;63(4):586–91.

[25] Hresko MT, Kasser JR. Physeal arrest about the knee associated with non-physeal fractures in the lower extremity. J Bone Joint Surg Am 1989;71(5):698–703.

[26] Kasser JR. Physeal bar resections after growth arrest about the knee. Clin Orthop Relat Res 1990;(255):68–74.

[27] Roberts JM. Operative treatment of fractures about the knee. Orthop Clin North Am 1990; 21(2):365–79.

[28] Burkhart SS, Peterson HA. Fractures of the proximal tibial epiphysis. J Bone Joint Surg Am 1979;61(7):996–1002.

[29] Aitken AP, Ingersoll RE. Fractures of the proximal tibial epiphyseal cartilage. J Bone Joint Surg Am 1956;38-A(4):787–96.

[30] Shelton WR, Canale ST. Fractures of the tibia through the proximal tibial epiphyseal cartilage. J Bone Joint Surg Am 1979;61(2):167–73.

[31] Ciszewski WA, Buschmann WR, Rudolph CN. Irreducible fracture of the proximal tibial physis in an adolescent. Orthop Rev 1989;18(8):891–3.

[32] Wood KB, Bradley JP, Ward WT. Pes anserinus interposition in a proximal tibial physeal fracture: a case report. Clin Orthop Relat Res 1991;(264):239–42.

[33] Watson-Jones R. Injuries of the knee. 4th edition. Baltimore (MD): Williams and Wilkins; 1955.

[34] Böhler L. The treatment of fractures. 5th edition. New York: Grune and Stratton; 1958.

[35] Hand WL, Hand CR, Dunn AW. Avulsion fractures of the tibial tubercle. J Bone Joint Surg Am 1971;53(8):1579–83.

[36] Mirbey J, Besancenot J, Chambers RT, et al. Avulsion fractures of the tibial tuberosity in the adolescent athlete: risk factors, mechanism of injury, and treatment. Am J Sports Med 1988;16(4):336–40.

[37] Ogden JA, Tross RB, Murphy MJ. Fractures of the tibial tuberosity in adolescents. J Bone Joint Surg Am 1980;62(2):205–15.

[38] Levi JH, Coleman CR. Fracture of the tibial tubercle. Am J Sports Med 1976;4:254–63.

[39] Christie MJ, Dvonch VM. Tibial tuberosity avulsion fracture in adolescents. J Pediatr Orthop 1981;1(4):391–4.

[40] Zionts LE. Fractures around the knee in children. J Am Acad Orthop Surg 2002;10(5): 345–55.

[41] Deliyannis SN. Avulsion of the tibial tuberosity: report of two cases. Injury 1973;4(4): 341–4.

[42] Gautier E, Ziran BH, Egger B, et al. Growth disturbances after injuries of the proximal tibial epiphysis. Arch Orthop Trauma Surg 1998;118(1–2):37–41.

[43] Pape JM, Goulet JA, Hensinger RN. Compartment syndrome complicating tibial tubercle avulsion. Clin Orthop Relat Res 1993;(295):201–4.

[44] Wiss DA, Schilz JL, Zionts L. Type III fractures of the tibial tubercle in adolescents. J Orthop Trauma 1991;5(4):475–9.

[45] Luhmann SJ. Acute traumatic knee effusions in children and adolescents. J Pediatr Orthop 2003;23(2):199–202.

[46] Skak SV, Jensen TT, Poulsen TD, et al. Epidemiology of knee injuries in children. Acta Orthop Scand 1987;58(1):78–81.

[47] Baxter MP, Wiley JJ. Fractures of the tibial spine in children: an evaluation of knee stability. J Bone Joint Surg Br 1988;70(2):228–30.

[48] Grönkvist H, Hirsch G, Johansson L. Fracture of the anterior tibial spine in children. J Pediatr Orthop 1984;4(4):465–8.

[49] Meyers MH, McKeever FM. Fracture of the intercondylar eminence of the tibia. J Bone Joint Surg Am 1970;52(8):1677–84.

[50] Willis RB, Blokker C, Stoll TM, et al. Long-term follow-up of anterior tibial eminence fractures. J Pediatr Orthop 1993;13(3):361–4.

[51] Kocher MS, Mandiga R, Klingele K, et al. Anterior cruciate ligament injury versus tibial spine fracture in the skeletally immature knee: a comparison of skeletal maturation and notch width index. J Pediatr Orthop 2004;24(2):185–8.

[52] Zaricznyj B. Avulsion fracture of the tibial eminence: treatment by open reduction and pinning. J Bone Joint Surg Am 1977;59(8):1111–4.

[53] Albright JC, Chambers H. Tibial eminence fractures. Philadelphia (PA): Saunders, Elsevier; 2006.

[54] Belman DA, Neviaser RJ. Transverse fracture of the patella in a child. J Trauma 1973; 13(10):917–8.

[55] Ray JM, Hendrix J. Incidence, mechanism of injury, and treatment of fractures of the patella in children. J Trauma 1992;32(4):464–7.

[56] Maguire JK, Canale ST. Fractures of the patella in children and adolescents. J Pediatr Orthop 1993;13(5):567–71.

[57] Houghton GR, Ackroyd CE. Sleeve fractures of the patella in children: a report of three cases. J Bone Joint Surg Br 1979;61-B(2):165–8.

[58] Nietosvaara Y, Aalto K, Kallio PE. Acute patellar dislocation in children: incidence and associated osteochondral fractures. J Pediatr Orthop 1994;14(4):513–5.

[59] Stefancin JJ, Parker RD. First-time traumatic patellar dislocation: a systematic review. Clin Orthop Relat Res 2007;455:93–101.

[60] Cash JD, Hughston JC. Treatment of acute patellar dislocation. Am J Sports Med 1988; 16(3):244–9.

[61] Rorabeck CH, Bobechko WP. Acute dislocation of the patella with osteochondral fracture: a review of eighteen cases. J Bone Joint Surg Br 1976;58(2):237–40.

[62] Stanitski CL, Paletta GA Jr. Articular cartilage injury with acute patellar dislocation in adolescents: arthroscopic and radiographic correlation. Am J Sports Med 1998;26(1):52–5.

[63] Oeppen RS, Connolly SA, Bencardino JT, et al. Acute injury of the articular cartilage and subchondral bone: a common but unrecognized lesion in the immature knee. AJR Am J Roentgenol 2004;182(1):111–7.

[64] Zaidi A, Babyn P, Astori I, et al. MRI of traumatic patellar dislocation in children. Pediatr Radiol 2006;36(11):1163–70.

[65] Sandmeier P, Burks RT, Bachus KN, et al. The effect of reconstruction of the medial patellofemoral ligament on patellar tracking. Am J Sports Med 2000;28:345–9.

[66] Conlan T, Garth WP Jr, Lemons JE. Evaluation of the medial soft-tissue restraints of the extensor mechanism of the knee. J Bone Joint Surg Am 1993;75(5):682–93.

[67] Desio SM, Burks RT, Bachus KN. Soft tissue restraints to lateral patellar translation in the human knee. Am J Sports Med 1998;26(1):59–65.

[68] Hautamaa PV, Fithian DC, Kaufman KR, et al. Medial soft tissue restraints in lateral patellar instability and repair. Clin Orthop Relat Res 1998;(349):174–82.

[69] Elias DA, White LM, Fithian DC. Acute lateral patellar dislocation at MR imaging: injury patterns of medial patellar soft-tissue restraints and osteochondral injuries of the inferome-dial patella. Radiology 2002;225(3):736–43.

[70] Avikainen VJ, Nikku RK, Seppanen-Lehmonen TK. Adductor magnus tenodesis for patellar dislocation: technique and preliminary results. Clin Orthop Relat Res 1993;(297):12–6.

[71] Nomura E. Classification of lesions of the medial patello-femoral ligament in patellar dislocation. Int Orthop 1999;23(5):260–3.

[72] Sallay PI, Poggi J, Speer KP, et al. Acute dislocation of the patella: a correlative pathoana-tomic study. Am J Sports Med 1996;24(1):52–60.

[73] Deie M, Ochi M, Sumen Y, et al. A long-term follow-up study after medial patellofemoral ligament reconstruction using the transferred semitendinosus tendon for patellar disloca-tion. Knee Surg Sports Traumatol Arthrosc 2005;13(7):522–8.

[74] Panagopoulos A, van Niekerk L, Triantafillopoulos IK. MPFL Reconstruction for recur-rent patella dislocation: a new surgical technique and review of the literature. Int J Sports Med Sep 18 2007, epub ahead of print.

[75] Souryal TO, Freeman TR. Intercondylar notch size and anterior cruciate ligament injuries in athletes: a prospective study. Am J Sports Med 1993;21(4):535–9.

[76] Kocher MS, DiCanzio J, Zurakowski D, et al. Diagnostic performance of clinical examina-tion and selective magnetic resonance imaging in the evaluation of intraarticular knee disorders in children and adolescents. Am J Sports Med 2001;29(3):292–6.

[77] Kocher MS, Micheli LJ, Zurakowski D, et al. Partial tears of the anterior cruciate ligament in children and adolescents. Am J Sports Med 2002;30(5):697–703.

[78] Stanitski CL, Harvell JC, Fu F. Observations on acute knee hemarthrosis in children and adolescents. J Pediatr Orthop 1993;13(4):506–10.

[79] Tanner J, Davies P. Clinical longitudinal standards for height and height velocity for North American children. J Pediatr 1985;107:317–29.

[80] Greulich W, Pyle S. Radiographic atlas of skeletal development of the hand and wrist. 2nd edition. Stanford (CA): Stanford University Press; 1959.

[81] Stanitski CL. Anterior cruciate ligament injury in the skeletally immature patient: diagnosis and treatment. J Am Acad Orthop Surg 1995;3(3):146–58.

[82] Aichroth PM, Patel DV, Zorrilla P. The natural history and treatment of rupture of the anterior cruciate ligament in children and adolescents: a prospective review. J Bone Joint Surg Br 2002;84(1):38–41.

[83] Graf BK, Lange RH, Fujisaki CK, et al. Anterior cruciate ligament tears in skeletally immature patients: meniscal pathology at presentation and after attempted conservative treatment. Arthroscopy 1992;8(2):229–33.

[84] Janarv PM, Nystrom A, Werner S, et al. Anterior cruciate ligament injuries in skeletally immature patients. J Pediatr Orthop 1996;16(5):673–7.

[85] McCarroll JR, Shelbourne KD, Porter DA, et al. Patellar tendon graft reconstruction for midsubstance anterior cruciate ligament rupture in junior high school athletes: an algorithm for management. Am J Sports Med 1994;22(4):478–84.

[86] Nottage WM, Matsuura PA. Management of complete traumatic anterior cruciate ligament tears in the skeletally immature patient: current concepts and review of the literature. Arthroscopy 1994;10(5):569–73.

[87] Pressman AE, Letts RM, Jarvis JG. Anterior cruciate ligament tears in children: an analysis of operative versus nonoperative treatment. J Pediatr Orthop 1997;17(4):505–11.

[88] DeLee JC, Curtis R. Anterior cruciate ligament insufficiency in children. Clin Orthop Relat Res 1983;(172):112–8.

[89] Engebretsen L, Svenningsen S, Benum P. Poor results of anterior cruciate ligament repair in adolescence. Acta Orthop Scand 1988;59(6):684–6.

[90] Aronowitz ER, Ganley TJ, Goode JR, et al. Anterior cruciate ligament reconstruction in adolescents with open physes. Am J Sports Med 2000;28(2):168–75.

[91] Micheli LJ, Rask B, Gerberg L. Anterior cruciate ligament reconstruction in patients who are prepubescent. Clin Orthop Relat Res 1999;(364):40–7.

[92] Guzzanti V, Falciglia F, Stanitski CL. Physeal-sparing intraarticular anterior cruciate ligament reconstruction in preadolescents. Am J Sports Med 2003;31(6):949–53.

[93] Anderson AF. Transepiphyseal replacement of the anterior cruciate ligament in skeletally immature patients: a preliminary report. J Bone Joint Surg Am 2003;85-A(7):1255–63.

[94] Kocher MS, Garg S, Micheli LJ. Physeal sparing reconstruction of the anterior cruciate ligament in skeletally immature prepubescent children and adolescents. J Bone Joint Surg Am 2005;87(11):2371–9.

[95] Andrews M, Noyes FR, Barber-Westin SD. Anterior cruciate ligament allograft reconstruction in the skeletally immature athlete. Am J Sports Med 1994;22(1):48–54.

[96] Bisson LJ, Wickiewicz T, Levinson M, et al. ACL reconstruction in children with open physes. Orthopedics 1998;21(6):659–63.

[97] Guzzanti V, Falciglia F, Stanitski CL. Preoperative evaluation and anterior cruciate ligament reconstruction technique for skeletally immature patients in Tanner stages 2 and 3. Am J Sports Med 2003;31(6):941–8.

[98] Lipscomb AB, Anderson AF. Tears of the anterior cruciate ligament in adolescents. J Bone Joint Surg Am 1986;68(1):19–28.

[99] Lo IK, Kirkley A, Fowler PJ, et al. The outcome of operatively treated anterior cruciate ligament disruptions in the skeletally immature child. Arthroscopy 1997;13(5):627–34.

[100] Janarv PM, Wikstrom B, Hirsch G. The influence of transphyseal drilling and tendon grafting on bone growth: an experimental study in the rabbit. J Pediatr Orthop 1998; 18(2):149–54.

[101] Seil R. ACL replacement in sheep with open physes: an evaluation of risk factors. ACL Study Group, Sardinia, Italy, May 30-June 3, 2004.

[102] Edwards TB, Greene CC, Baratta RV, et al. The effect of placing a tensioned graft across open growth plates: a gross and histologic analysis. J Bone Joint Surg Am 2001;83-A(5): 725–34.

[103] Shelbourne KD, Gray T, Wiley BV. Results of transphyseal anterior cruciate ligament reconstruction using patellar tendon autograft in Tanner stage 3 or 4 adolescents with clearly open growth plates. Am J Sports Med 2004;32(5):1218–22.

[104] Fuchs R, Wheatley W, Uribe JW, et al. Intra-articular anterior cruciate ligament reconstruction using patellar tendon allograft in the skeletally immature patient. Arthroscopy 2002;18(8):824–8.

[105] Unwin A. ACL Reconstruction in the immature skeleton. ACL Study Group, Sardinia, Italy, May 30-June 3, 2004.

[106] Kocher MS, Saxon HS, Hovis WD, et al. Management and complications of anterior cruciate ligament injuries in skeletally immature patients: survey of the Herodicus Society and the ACL Study Group. J Pediatr Orthop 2002;22(4):452–7.

[107] Koman JD, Sanders JO. Valgus deformity after reconstruction of the anterior cruciate ligament in a skeletally immature patient: a case report. J Bone Joint Surg Am 1999; 81(5):711–5.

[108] Smith AD, Tao SS. Knee injuries in young athletes. Clin Sports Med 1995;14(3):629–50.

[109] Jones RE, Henley MB, Francis P. Nonoperative management of isolated grade III collateral ligament injury in high school football players. Clin Orthop Relat Res 1986;(213):137–40.

[110] Sankar WN, Wells L, Sennett BJ, et al. Combined anterior cruciate ligament and medial collateral ligament injuries in adolescents. J Pediatr Orthop 2006;26(6):733–6.

[111] Chen FS, Rokito AS, Pitman MI. Acute and chronic posterolateral rotatory instability of the knee. J Am Acad Orthop Surg 2000;8(2):97–110.

[112] Clark CR, Ogden JA. Development of the menisci of the human knee joint: morphological changes and their potential role in childhood meniscal injury. J Bone Joint Surg Am 1983; 65(4):538–47.

[113] Andrish JT. Meniscal injuries in children and adolescents: diagnosis and management. J Am Acad Orthop Surg 1996;4(5):231–7.

[114] Iobst CA, Stanitski CL. Acute knee injuries. Clin Sports Med 2000;19(4):621–35.

[115] Stanitski CL. Correlation of arthroscopic and clinical examinations with magnetic resonance imaging findings of injured knees in children and adolescents. Am J Sports Med 1998;26(1):2–6.

[116] Luhmann SJ, Schootman M, Gordon JE, et al. Magnetic resonance imaging of the knee in children and adolescents: its role in clinical decision-making. J Bone Joint Surg Am 2005; 87(3):497–502.

[117] King AG. Meniscal lesions in children and adolescents: a review of the pathology and clinical presentation. Injury 1983;15(2):105–8.

[118] Ritchie DM. Meniscectomy in children. Aust N Z J Surg 1966;35(3):239–41.

[119] Asik M, Atalar AC. Failed resorption of bioabsorbable meniscus repair devices. Knee Surg Sports Traumatol Arthrosc 2002;10(5):300–4.

[120] Ellermann A, Siebold R, Buelow JU, et al. Clinical evaluation of meniscus repair with a bioabsorbable arrow: a 2- to 3-year follow-up study. Knee Surg Sports Traumatol Arthrosc 2002;10(5):289–93.

[121] Miller MD, Kline AJ, Gonzales J, et al. Pitfalls associated with FasT-Fix meniscal repair. Arthroscopy 2002;18(8):939–43.

[122] Sims WF, Simonian PT. Delayed degradation of bioabsorbable meniscal fixators. Arthroscopy 2001;17(3):E11.

[123] Edelson RH, Katchis SD, Parker RD. Complications of meniscus repair. Oper Tech Sports Med 1994;2:208–16.

[124] Committee on Complications of the Arthroscopy Association of North America. Complications in arthroscopy: the knee and other joints. Arthroscopy 1986;2:253–8.

[125] Hergenroeder AC. Prevention of sports injuries. Pediatrics 1998;101(6):1057–63.

[126] Goldstein JD, Berger PE, Windler GE, et al. Spine injuries in gymnasts and swimmers: an epidemiologic investigation. Am J Sports Med 1991;19(5):463–8.

[127] Hewett TE, Lindenfeld TN, Riccobene JV, et al. The effect of neuromuscular training on the incidence of knee injury in female athletes: a prospective study. Am J Sports Med 1999;27(6):699–706.

[128] Brenner JS. Overuse injuries, overtraining, and burnout in child and adolescent athletes. Pediatrics 2007;119(6):1242–5.

[129] Fox K, Goudas M, Biddle S, et al. Children's task and ego goal profiles in sport. Br J Educ Psychol 1994;64(Pt 2):253–61.

ELSEVIER
SAUNDERS

Phys Med Rehabil Clin N Am
19 (2008) 347–371

PHYSICAL MEDICINE
AND REHABILITATION
CLINICS OF
NORTH AMERICA

Common Injuries of the Foot and Ankle in the Child and Adolescent Athlete

Gerard A. Malanga, MD[a,b,c,*],
Jose A. Ramirez – Del Toro, MD[d]

[a]Department of Physical Medicine and Rehabilitation, University of Medicine and Dentistry,
New Jersey Medical School, 30 Bergen Street, Newark, NJ 07101, USA
[b]Mountainside Hospital, 1 Bay Avenue, Montclair, NJ 07042, USA
[c]Department of Rehabilitation Medicine, Pain Management Center, Overlook Hospital,
MAC II Building, Suite B110, 11 Overlook Road, Summit, NJ 07091, USA
[d]Sports Medicine and Spinal Intervention, New Jersey Sports Medicine Institute,
Montclair, NJ, USA

One of the most commonly injured parts of the body in adolescent athletes is the foot and ankle. It can account for up to 30% of visits to sports medicine clinics [1,2]. Ankle sprains alone account for 10% of all injuries seen in the emergency room [3]. Different sports can cause different types of injuries in the foot and ankle. In basketball, for example, foot and ankle injuries have been shown to account for 44% to 45% of all injuries in adolescent athletes, and in the adolescent football player, the foot and ankle make up 13% to 16% of all injuries [4–6]. Most of these injuries are lateral ankle sprains. Long distance runners report foot injuries as the most common injury they sustain [7–9], and adolescent runners are susceptible to overuse type of injuries [10]. Young dancers and gymnasts also have a high percentage of foot and ankle injuries, with their specific sports mechanics often predisposing to acute fractures and fatigue fractures [11,12]. It is important that physicians feel comfortable with the common injuries that can occur in the foot and ankle and be able to identify these injuries in the young athlete.

When treating young athletes, physicians must keep in mind the anatomic developmental differences that exist between the skeletally mature and the skeletally immature foot and ankle. These anatomic differences predispose young athletes to an entirely different set of injuries than the adult athlete. A thorough understanding of general bony, ligamentous, and muscular

* Corresponding author.
E-mail address: gmalanga@pol.net (G.A. Malanga).

anatomy of the foot and ankle is also valuable to be able to accurately devise a differential diagnosis based on symptom location.

In this article we first address, define, and explain the types of injuries and injury patterns germane to the developing skeletally immature athlete. Next, before discussing all the common injuries, we present a brief anatomic review of the basic bony anatomy of the ankle and foot for reference purposes. In an anatomically oriented fashion, we outline the most common injuries noted in the pediatric and adolescent ankle and foot. There is emphasis on history, physical examination, diagnosis, and basic treatment guidelines. We look at the lateral ankle, the medial and anterior ankle, and the hindfoot, midfoot, and forefoot.

Injury patterns in the developing athlete

The presence of a growth plate, known as the physis or the epiphyseal plate, is a major difference in developing musculoskeletal structures that is not seen in the fully mature skeleton. The long bones of children contain the physis between the metaphysis and the epiphysis (Fig. 1). Bone is laid down for growth in the physis; however, this area is not a stable and strong area because it is constantly changing and remodeling. There is relative weakness at the growth plate and its surrounding bony structures as compared with the ligamentous structures about the pediatric and adolescent foot and ankle [1]. The epiphyseal plate is also less resistant to shear and tensile forces than the adjacent bony structures [13]. In adults, the opposite is true. The bone is strong, and the sites of injuries are in the ligamentous and muscular structures because they are the weaker points [14]. For example, where an inversion rollover injury would cause ligamentous injury in an adult, it is much more likely to cause injury at the growth plate in a child, possibly leading to a fracture of the physis or epiphyseal plate.

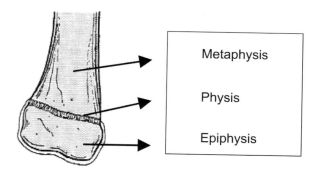

Fig. 1. A pictorial depiction of the metaphysis, physis, and epiphysis of the developing bone. (*Adapted from* Canale ST. Physeal injuries. In: Green NE, Swiontkowski MF, editors. Skeletal trauma in children. 3rd edition. Philadelphia: WB Saunders; 2003. p. 17–56; with permission.)

Generally, the injuries seen in skeletally immature athletes can be divided into three main categories: (1) injuries related to growth, (2) overuse injuries, and (3) acute presentations [13–15]. Pain related to growth stems from bony coalitions or accessory ossification centers that may be abnormally developing. Overuse injuries include osteochondroses, apophysitis, and stress fractures. Acute injuries include the full spectrum of ligament, tendon, and muscle injuries and acute fractures. Epiphyseal injuries can be from overuse and acute traumatic events. An overview is provided, and a more comprehensive discussion of the specific injuries follows.

Growth-related problems: coalitions and accessory ossicles

A coalition is a connection or fusion of two or more bones. It can be a bony, cartilaginous, or fibrous connection [16–18]. Endochondral ossification is the formation of new bone from tissues such as cartilage, and there are two ossification centers in bone. The primary ossification center is located in the diaphysis, and the secondary ossification center is the physis (physeal plate, epiphyseal plate, or growth plate) located between the diaphysis and the epiphysis [19]. Because coalitions are composed of bony, fibrous, or cartilaginous tissues, they can act as their own ossification centers. When they ossify, they become painful where the tissues are placed under stress, particularly in highly active adolescent athletes [1,16]. The most common coalitions are talocalcaneal and calcaneonavicular coalitions.

Accessory ossicles are separate ossification centers located extrachondrally. They differ from coalitions because they do not form a connection between two bones but exist at the end of certain bones. Accessory ossicles usually appear at age 8 to 10 years and usually fuse approximately 1 year after their formation. When they do not fuse, they become symptomatic [16]. The most common sites for accessory ossification center formation are at the posterior talus, known as os trigonum, the medial malleolus, and the navicular. The navicular ossification center sometimes can form an entirely new bone known as an accessory navicular.

Overuse injuries: apophysitis and osteochondroses

Overuse injuries in sports have been defined as chronic injuries related to constant repetitive stress without adequate recovery time [20]. The cause is believed to be repetitive application of a submaximal stress to normal tissue that overwhelms the normal repair process [15,20–22]. These types of injuries can develop in one of three ways in the adolescent athlete population [20]. First, they can occur in athletes who increase their activity level rapidly without adequate training, as in individuals who begin preseason workouts without having practiced the sport for long periods. Second, they can occur in ill-prepared children who lack good mechanical sport-specific skills. Third, they can occur in vigorous athletes who do not provide their body with adequate rest from activity. Overuse injuries in the adolescent foot and ankle can present at (1) the insertion of the tendon to the bone, which is known as the apophysis, (2) the articular cartilage, which causes what is known as an osteochondrosis injury, and (3) the growing bone itself, which presents as a stress fracture [15,23].

The apophysis is the area of junction between a tendon/musculotendinous unit and the epiphysis. Sometimes these sites of attachment also cross the physeal growth plate. These areas are constantly placed under stress from repeated contractions and traction at the site, which can lead to irritation or inflammation at the physis, known as apophysitis [1,24]. The most common sites for the occurrence of apophysitis that we discuss are at the calcaneus (Sever's disease) and at the base of the fifth metatarsal (Iselin's disease).

Osteochondroses refer to lesions thought to be related to overuse, although it also believed that osteonecrosis may play a role in their development [15,25]. What is known is that they are lesions of the ossification centers that eventually undergo recalcification [1]. The two most common lesions that we discuss are osteochondrosis of the tarsal navicular, known as Kohler's disease, and osteochondrosis of the second or third metatarsal heads, known as Freiberg's infarction. It is worth noting that an osteochondral lesion of the talus—a complication of lateral ankle sprains—is not technically considered an osteochondrosis or overuse injury, although the pathology is located in the talar dome articular cartilage. These injuries can occur with up to 6.5% of ankle sprains and are discussed as a chronic presentation of an acute injury [26].

Overuse injuries: stress fractures

A stress fracture can occur anywhere in the pediatric and adolescent foot and ankle and is believed to be the ultimate overuse injury [16,27]. It has been referred to as a process that leads to fatigue or insufficiency failure of bone that occurs when the bone's reparative abilities have been surpassed [13,16,28] and the bone is unable to withstand chronic repetitive submaximal loads [29]. These injuries account for up to 15% of all athletic injuries in young athletes [30]. Stress fractures are most commonly seen in adolescent runners [10,20] but are associated with almost any sport in which repetitive running and cutting movements occur [29,31].

Multiple risk factors exist for the development of stress fractures, including sudden increases in training, poor mechanics, improper or worn-out footwear, young age, and poor nutrition with low bone mineral density [1,20,32–36]. Recently there has been an increase in stress fractures in young female athletes, and a connection has been made between anorexia, amenorrhea, and osteoporosis and the incidence of stress fractures [10,15]. This population is also at increased risk. In the foot and ankle, stress fractures can occur anywhere, but the most common sites are the metatarsals and the tibial diaphysis [20]. Stress fractures of the medial and lateral malleolus can occur in adolescents but are more common in adult athletes. Tarsal navicular stress fractures are also common and difficult to treat.

In a study on military recruits, the occurrence of stress fractures was most prominent in the first month of training, when the increased training and repetitive loads led to increased osteoclastic activity and the osteoblastic activity had not caught up with the remodeling process [36]. Research indicated that bone mineral content increased after 14 weeks of training, possibly acting to prevent continued occurrence of stress fractures. This finding argues in favor of evidence that accelerated bone remodeling during the time when overuse is occurring is directly associated with stress fracture development.

Patients who have stress fractures commonly present with insidious onset of pain that worsens with increased activity and dissipates once the activity is stopped [37]. There is usually a history of an increase in the amount of training that coincides with the onset of symptoms; therefore, they are thought to be overuse injuries [13]. On physical examination, palpation can recreate symptoms depending on the location of the fracture. There may be point tenderness with no history of acute discrete traumatic event.

Radiographs often do not show evidence of the fractures initially [38]. It has been reported that only 10% of initial radiographs showed abnormalities [29,39]. It may take 3 to 4 weeks for the reactive process associated with stress fractures to become visible on radiographs, and often the first sign of this reactive process is subperiosteal new bone formation [13]. Results of radiographs also may remain normal if athletic activity is decreased [38]. In cases in which the diagnosis is suspected, a three-phase bone scan is most sensitive in detecting the stress fracture [38].

Proper treatment of stress fractures, as with most overuse injuries, requires a period of 2 to 4 weeks of relative rest, with temporary cessation of running. Usually partial weight bearing is tolerated, unless the symptoms are present during walking and light activity. During this period of modified rest, the osteoblastic activity catches up and restores balance [1]. It is important to maintain some level of cardiopulmonary fitness program, including non–land-based training, such as pool activities or cycling. Progression to running depends on symptoms and is individualized. Please note that these specifications do not apply to navicular stress fractures, whose management is somewhat different.

Acute problems: epiphyseal fracture classification

Acute fractures of the ends of long bones in children are common because of the relative weakness of the epiphysis in relation to the surrounding soft tissues. The literature is full of different ways to attempt classify these fractures. Some systems attempt to define the position of the foot with relation to the leg, whereas other systems attempt to define the fracture patterns in terms of the direction of the force placed on the leg [15,40–45]. These systems can be useful, but unless one is communicating with specialists, there is not good communication regarding the injury.

One system that is widely used by specialists and primary care physicians to communicate about growth plate fractures is the Salter-Harris classification system (Fig. 2) [46]. It is essential to have a grasp on this way of referring to physeal plate fractures. This system not only gives an anatomic and radiologic way of describing these injuries unique to the child and adolescent population but also provides useful prognostic implications that may affect treatment and the potential for growth disturbances [47,48]. For example, Salter-Harris type I fractures of the distal fibula are rarely complicated by growth arrests, whereas Salter-Harris type II fractures of the distal tibia do have a significant incidence of growth arrest [14,49].

Salter-Harris fractures of the foot and ankle most commonly are seen in the distal tibia and distal fibula and the phalanges [15]. The most common acute injury of the adolescent foot and ankle is a Salter-Harris type I

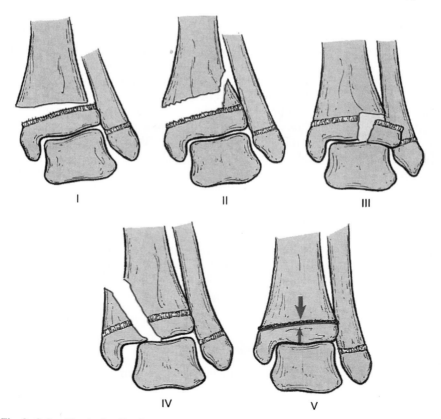

Fig. 2. Salter-Harris classification of physeal injury. (*Adapted from* Canale ST. Physeal injuries. In: Green NE, Swiontkowski MF, editors. Skeletal trauma in children. 3rd edition. Philadelphia: WB Saunders; 2003. p. 17–56; with permission.)

fracture of the distal fibula, which has been called the childhood equivalent of the lateral ankle sprain in skeletally mature patients [14]. Type I Salter-Harris fractures are confined to the growth plate, and they do not involve either the metaphysis or the epiphysis. Salter-Harris type II fractures involve the growth plate and usually a margin of the metaphysis. The epiphysis is not involved. These fractures are by far the most common types of growth plate fractures seen [15]. Salter-Harris type III fractures occur when a fracture line extends vertically or obliquely through a section of the epiphysis and proximally to reach the growth plate. In these fractures, the metaphysis is not involved. Salter-Harris type IV fractures extend vertically through the epiphysis, into the physeal growth plate, and into the metaphysis. Type V Salter-Harris injuries usually result from a compressive or crushing force. They are rare and often have no radiographic abnormality.

Treatment of physeal growth plate fractures depends on multiple factors, including the location of the injury, the Salter-Harris classification, the age of the child, and the potential pitfalls and complications of each injury [48]. The age of the child is particularly important because the growth plate may be fully open if the child is young or may be closing if the child is older. In the latter case, there is less concern for growth arrest and significant leg-length discrepancy because there is likely little growth remaining. If the child is younger, premature physeal closure is a concerning complication. These fractures usually heal within 4 to 6 weeks [50].

General guidelines state that for Salter-Harris type I and II fractures, closed reduction and cast immobilization with a short leg walking cast for 3 to 4 weeks are usually the initial treatments of choice, unless there is any level of displacement of the fracture, in which case maintenance of reduction must be undertaken, sometimes necessitating wire placement [14,15,50]. The patient is followed with serial radiographs to ensure that no complications occur. These fractures have been thought to be fairly uncomplicated. Recently, however, studies illuminated that premature physeal closure may be more common than previously thought [51]. Salter-Harris types III and IV always require closed reduction, but if their displacement is more than 2 mm, usually open reduction with internal fixation is favored. Two specific kinds of Salter-Harris fractures are presented later in this article: the Tillaux fracture and the triplane fracture.

Brief anatomic review of foot and ankle

The most pertinent bony anatomy is as follows: the ankle joint is a synovial joint composed of three bones: the tibia, fibula, and talus (Fig. 3). The proximal articulating surface of the ankle is composed of the concave end of the distal tibia and its medial malleolus and the lateral fibular malleolus [52]. This proximal articulating surface extends more distally in its posterior and lateral borders. It forms a mortise-type shape into which the distal articulating surface of the ankle—the talus—articulates; there is inherent stability in

A

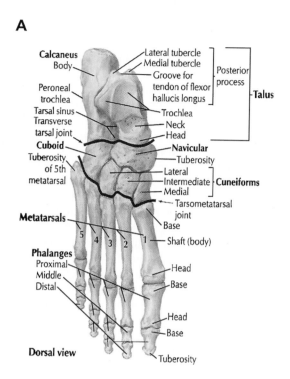

B

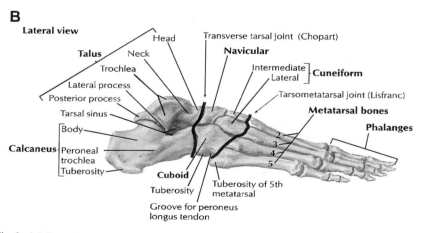

Fig. 3. (*A*) Dorsal views of the foot and ankle bony anatomy. (*B*) Lateral view of the ankle and foot bony anatomy. (*Reprinted with permission from* Netter Anatomy Illustration Collection, © Elsevier Inc. All rights reserved.)

this type of formation. The hindfoot is composed of the talus and the calcaneous bones. The articulation between these two is the subtalar joint. The midfoot is composed of the navicular, the cuboid, and the three cuneiforms: medial, intermediate, and lateral. The articulation of the distal talus and calcaneus with the proximal navicular and cuboid bones forms the midtarsal joint. The forefoot is composed of the five metatarsals and the 14 phalanges. The articulation of the three cuneiforms and the cuboid distally with the proximal metatarsals forms Lisfranc's joint. Note the following three articulations: (1) the talus with the calcaneous (ie, subtalar joint), (2) the talus with the navicular, and (3) the calcaneous with the cuboid. (Articulations 2 and 3 are known as the transverse tarsal joints.) These three joints are collectively known as the three-joint complex, and they are crucial structures for the dissipation of forces throughout the ankle and foot during gait mechanics [53].

Anatomic location of injury presentations

Lateral ankle

Acute injuries
Lateral ankle sprain. In the lateral ankle, developmental or overuse type of injuries are uncommon. The possibility exists of an ossification center in the fibular region or peroneal tendonitis overuse issues, but they are rare. The most common predominant injury in a child's lateral ankle, after the Salter-Harris type I physeal fracture of the distal fibula, which was discussed earlier, is the lateral ankle sprain. It is less common in younger children, because they are more apt to injure the fibular physeal plate for the aforementioned reason that the epiphysis and the growth plate are inherently weak points in the childhood ankle. In more mature adolescents, however, the bone is stronger and the growth plate is ossifying and closing, so injuries of the ligaments are common [14].

The main function of the anterior talofibular ligament (ATFL) and calcaneofibular ligament (CFL) complex is the prevention of excessive lateral or varus translation of the ankle [52]. The typical mechanism of a lateral ankle sprain occurs when the ankle is subjected to an inversion and internal rotation force while in plantarflexion [54,55]. The ATFL is the first ligament injured, and the CFL is also at risk of injury, although it is more likely injured if the ankle is in dorsiflexion. One common method of injury involves landing on another athlete's foot while coming down from a jump. Patients complain of immediate pain and, depending on the severity of the sprain, may have swelling over the area. Depending on the severity of the injury, the patient may be unable to bear weight on it.

Physical examination usually reveals tenderness over the ATFL or the CFL with palpation. There may be ecchymosis and swelling and tenderness with active and passive range of motion of the ankle. Two maneuvers can be performed to assess the integrity of the ATFL and the CFL, respectively: the anterior draw test and the talar tilt or varus stress test [56]. A positive anterior draw is more than 3 to 5 mm difference in anterior displacement of the ankle in side-to-side comparisons. Results of the talar tilt test are positive when there is more than 23° of angulation or more than 10° of difference side to side. The specificity and sensitivity for the anterior draw are 80%–94% and 74%–84% respectiviely. These have not been reported for the talar tilt [57]. Severity of injury is usually based on a three-point grading system. Grade 1 sprains are mild and involve a partial tear of the ATFL with intact CFL. There is usually tenderness to palpation, but only mild swelling. The anterior draw and the talar tilt tests usually have negative results. Grade 2 sprains are moderate and involve complete tears of the ATFL and mild tears of the CFL. There is diffuse swelling and ecchymosis and a large anterior shift on the anterior draw test. The talar tilt test usually has negative results. Grade 3 sprains are severe and involve tears of the ATFL and the CFL, with both tests producing positive results [58].

Radiographic imaging in lateral ankle sprain-type injuries in children is somewhat controversial. In adults, the Ottawa Ankle Rules (OAR) were devised by Stiell and colleagues because too many ankle radiographs were being obtained in emergency departments [59,60]. The sensitivity of the OAR is 100% and the specificity is 40% for the detection of ankle fractures. If a patient does not meet the rules, then no imaging is necessary [60]. With OAR, however, all patients were older than 18 years. In children younger than18 years, there may be issues of weak growth plates and the possibility of physeal fractures. Some physicians have argued that nearly all children with ankle pain merit an evaluation with plain radiographs to assess the integrity of the bony structures and to look for congenital or developmental anomalies [61]. Clark and colleagues [59] tried to apply the OAR to children. They came up with a sensitivity of 83%, specificity of 50%, positive predictive value of 28%, and negative predictive value (NPV) of 93% and concluded that the OAR could not be applied to children.

In another prospective study, Boutis and colleagues [62] used a specific set of physical examination parameters for children and adolescents with ankle sprains who presented to the emergency department. Their low-risk clinical examination was defined as isolated tenderness, with or without edema or ecchymosis of the distal fibula below the level of the joint line and/or over the adjacent lateral ligaments (ATFL, posterior talofibular ligament, CFL). All other findings on examination were believed to be high risk. They stratified all injuries into low risk and high risk based on their examination and obtained radiographic views on all subjects to confirm their findings. It is worth noting that the diagnoses that they considered to be low risk included sprains, contusions, lateral talar avulsion fractures, and fractures of the distal fibula, including nondisplaced Salter-Harris I and II and epiphyseal avulsion fractures. These fractures were considered low risk because they are stable injuries that carry excellent prognosis and their management is usually based on maximizing comfort, according to the authors. All other fractures were classified as high risk. They found that none of the 381 enrolled children with low-risk examinations had high-risk fractures (sensitivity 100% and NPV 100%). They concomitantly applied the OAR to all children and analyzed how the OAR would have fared as far as limiting the number of radiographs. They found that with their low-risk examination, 63% of radiographs could have been omitted, whereas only a 12% reduction in radiographs would have occurred with the OAR [62].

Proper treatment is essential for adequate return to competition in youth sports and to prevent future negative sequelae associated with improperly managed ankle sprains [63,64]. Some guidelines have been set forth in the literature, but much of the basic concepts are the same [65–67]. It also has been noted that early mobilization may promote better healing by producing better orientation of the collagen fibers when compared with an immobilized joint [1,68]. The basic guidelines of the PRICE acronym are used at first: protection, rest, ice, compression, and elevation. Patients may bear weight as tolerated with protective support and crutches. As patients progress from the acute to subacute phase of the injury and their pain at rest decreases, the goal should be to attempt to increase pain-free range of motion. Cardiovascular fitness comprised of upper extremity or non–weight-bearing aerobic work also should be undertaken. As the swelling and pain diminish, progressive weight bearing should be performed. Strengthening also should begin to progress from isometric to isotonic and isokinetic exercises based on patient symptomatology. Proprioceptive training also should be initiated to improve neuromuscular signaling and decrease future ankle instability. Once patients reach full range of motion with minimal or no pain on vigorous activity, sport-specific functional progression should occur [65]. The overall goal of the rehabilitative program should be to return athletes to full strength and range of motion and attempt to decrease the recurrence rates of sprains with improved proprioceptive neuromuscular control and confidence in the ankle.

Talar osteochondral defects. Talar dome injuries are common complications of lateral ankle sprains and occur in up to 6.5% of cases [26]. The mechanism by which the lesions develop is still not fully elucidated, but the belief is that poor healing after an ankle sprain or other ankle trauma leads to poor circulation to the subchondral bone of the talus, which in turn leads to these focal lesions of almost necrotic bone fragments [69,70]. The injury is most common in the second decade of life, and up to 100% of the lateral lesions are believed to be from previous ankle sprains or trauma, whereas 64% of patients with medial lesions had a history of trauma [69,71].

The typical history is an adolescent athlete with ankle pain and either a persistent effusion or the occurrence of intermittent swelling of the joint. There may be a history of the ankle catching or locking and some instability and episodes of giving way [72]. Inevitably, further probing detects a history of ankle sprains at some point in the athletic career of the patient and usually one that was not properly rehabilitated. Along the same lines, when an ankle sprain does not respond to 6 to 8 weeks of conservative treatment, then talar dome osteochondral lesions must be highly suspected and ruled out [72].

Radiographs often demonstrate the lesions fairly clearly, particularly with mortise views. Berndt and Harty [73] developed a classification system for these lesions based on radiographic appearance, which helps to guide management of the lesions. Stage I lesions show localized trabecular compression. Stage II lesions are incompletely separated fragments. Stage III lesions are undetached, undisplaced fragments. Stage IV lesions demonstrate a displaced or inverted fragment floating free within the joint. When radiographs do not demonstrate the lesions but clinical suspicion remains high, MRI can serve as a valuable tool for diagnosis. MRI helps to distinguish among stable lesions, loose in situ lesions, and loose lesions [74]. Stable lesions correlate with Berndt and Harty stage I and II lesions that have healed. Loose in situ and loose lesions correlate with stages III and IV lesions in the Berndt and Harty classification system.

Treatment for the stage I, stage II, and medial stage III lesions is nonoperative, short leg cast immobilization with limited or non–weight bearing for 6 to 8 weeks, whereas surgery is indicated for lateral sided stage III lesions and all stage IV lesions [75]. The authors believe that the best treatment for this lesion is prevention of its occurrence, which may be accomplished if a comprehensive therapy and rehabilitative program for lateral ankle sprains (much like the one outlined previously) is performed, with a focus on early mobilization, range-of-motion training, proprioceptive training, and progressive strengthening.

Medial and anterior ankle

Growth-related problems
Medial malleolus ossification center. The medial malleolus ossification center is present in all children. It usually appears at 1 to 2 years of age and closes by age 12 [16]. This center occasionally persists into adulthood but is usually asymptomatic. It becomes a problem in adolescents when they are overly active athletically [16,76]. The usual presentation is pain, point tenderness, and swelling over the medial malleolus without a significant history of trauma or any acute injury to the area. Anteroposterior radiographs of the ankle demonstrate an irregular ossification center with an associated ossicle [14,16,76]. Treatment includes rest from athletic activities with at least 3 to 6 weeks of short leg cast immobilization [76]. If no improvement occurs with this regimen, surgery for removal of the ossicle may be indicated.

Overuse injuries
Anterior ankle impingement syndrome. Bony anterior ankle impingement is a painful condition seen in many young athletes. It is an irritation of the

periosteum on the talar neck that leads to bony exostosis, which in turn leads to impingement [14,16]. It is commonly seen in athletes, such as ballet dancers and gymnasts, who are constantly in extremes of dorsiflexion; it is considered an overuse type of injury. Patients present with pain in the anterior ankle and a history of participating vigorously in a sport or activity that lends itself to repeated dorsiflexion moments. Pain is usually exacerbated by dorsiflexion movements, such as pliés in ballet dancers. Dancers often complain of limited dorsiflexion range of motion in the affected ankle, which may be noted during the examination [11]. Radiographs demonstrate an anterior tibial or talar neck osteophyte that has developed from the exostosis from overuse [11]. Conservative treatment consists of stretching of the Achilles tendon to attempt to improve range of motion and strengthening of the dorsiflexors [14]. Rest from activity and icing may help. According to one author, however, by the time an adolescent dancer presents with this problem, it usually cannot be solved with conservative measures, and a surgical excision of the osteophyte is needed [11]. The dancer usually can return to full plié position in 3 to 4 months if adequate postsurgical rehabilitation is conducted.

Acute injuries

Tillaux fractures. A Tillaux fracture is the most common Salter-Harris type III fracture seen in adolescents [14,15]. It is an isolated fracture of the distal anterolateral tibial physis. During normal development, the medial and posterior tibial physeal plates close first, and then the anterolateral areas close. This fracture occurs late in the teen years in the period when the medial and posterior plates have closed and the anterior growth plate is still open [15]. The most common mechanism of injury is a forceful external rotation-type injury. As the ankle is stressed medially, the pull of the anterior tibiofibular ligament results in an avulsion fracture of the anterolateral aspect of the distal tibial epiphysis over the area of the physeal plate that is still not ossified [15]. Because that physeal plate is not yet closed, it remains a structural weak link. The medial and posterior parts of the epiphysis are not affected because the growth plate already has ossified and closed and it is not a weak point any more [15]. Patients present with anterior ankle pain and swelling in the setting of an external rotation trauma. Radiographs reveal a vertical line that extends from the anterior ankle joint proximally through the epiphysis to the growth plate. Treatment depends on the amount of displacement of the growth plate. If it is less than 2 mm, then closed reduction and a short leg walking cast for 4 to 6 weeks are favored, as noted in the discussion on Salter-Harris fractures. Fracture displacements that are more than 2 mm necessitate open reduction and internal fixation [15,77].

Triplane fractures. Triplane fractures represent yet another type of fracture of the distal anterior tibial epiphysis and physeal growth plate. These fractures are similar to Tillaux fractures in two main ways. First, they normally occur in the period when the anterolateral plate is still open and other areas of the distal tibial growth plate have closed. The pattern of what has and has not been ossified is what determines the extent of the injury [78]. Second, the triplane fracture occurs from external rotation forces of the ankle, which cause shearing and avulsion. Some authors speculate that plantarflexion may contribute to their occurrence and to their irregularity in presentation and on radiographs [79]. They differ from Tillaux fractures in that the extent of involvement of the terminal bone is greater and involves the metaphysis, physis, and epiphysis. Triplane fractures are more difficult to diagnose on plain radiographs because their full extent may not be seen on regular views of the ankle. CT scans usually delineate the lesion well [15]. Treatment is same as for Tillaux fractures, and if surgery is performed, adequate visualization of all fracture fragments is paramount to successful outcomes [15,80].

Hindfoot

Growth-related problems

Talocalcaneal coalition. Tarsal coalitions are fusions of two or more of the tarsal bones [1,16]. The incidence of coalitions may be as high as 1% to 3% in the population and are bilateral 50% of the time [1,81]. The most common tarsal coalitions are the talocalcaneal and the calcaneonavicular coalitions, which account for 90% of all coalitions [1]. The subtalar joint, the talocalcaneal articulation, and the calcaneocuboid articulation form the three-joint complex. This complex is responsible for many foot motions during the gait cycle. The presence of a talocalcaneal and calcaneonavicular coalition severely affects the motion at the three-joint complex [81].

The typical presentation of a painful coalition occurs in the developing mid- to late teenage athlete who participates in vigorous activity. It is then that the presence of the congenital coalition first becomes evident. Increasing activity, combined with maturing ossification, leads to motion alteration and pain. Pain is usually located vaguely around the ankle based on the location of the coalition and based on which motion segment in the three-joint complex is mostly affected. There may or may not be a history of previous lateral ankle sprains [81]. Physical examination reveals findings associated with decreased motion of the hindfoot. The hindfoot is held in rigid valgus, and there is absence of heel varus on tiptoes. There is often rigid flat foot, and peroneal tightness and spasticity can be seen in their attempts to overcome the rigid flat foot. Pain is also present with foot inversion [1,81,82].

Radiographically, the talocalcaneal coalition is difficult to identify on plain radiographs, although the calcaneonavicular one is usually well visualized. CT is considered the gold standard imaging modality for the diagnosis of tarsal coalitions, however [83]. Treatment initially targets symptom control. If athletic activity worsens the symptoms, then the activity should be decreased or temporarily stopped. Orthotics can help control mild symptoms.

Cast immobilization for 6 weeks in a short leg walking cast is indicated, particularly with painful and stiff joints [81]. Failure of conservative therapy is marked by continued pain and inability to participate in sports. Surgical options include excision of the coalition, calcaneal osteotomy, and arthrodesis of the joint [1,81].

Os trigonum. A normal ossification center can often be located at the posterior aspect of the talus. It usually appears at 9 to 12 years of age and fuses 1 year after its appearance. When it does not ossify, an ossicle develops, which is known as the os trigonum [16]. It has been reported to be present in as much as 10% of the population, and it is usually unilateral [16,84]. It becomes symptomatic in young athletes who perform repeated ankle plantarflexion, such as ballet dancers, gymnasts, and ice skaters. One of the mechanisms by which it is believed to cause pain is from mechanical impingement of the posterior talus between the posterior tibia and the calcaneous when the foot is in plantarflexion [16,84]. The presentation is an active athlete who has pain in the posterolateral ankle that is reproducible on palpation and active plantarflexion. The os trigonum is usually seen on lateral plain radiographs as an ossicle located posterior to the calcaneus. It has been recommended that plantarflexion views also be obtained for verification [16]. Treatment is conservative. Plantarflexion must be avoided as much as possible. If the pain continues with resumption of the athletic activity, then surgical resection may be indicated. Some authors recommend early resection in competitive young athletes as the best way to resolve the symptomatology and expedite return to play safely [85].

Overuse injuries
Sever's apophysitis. Apophyses are bony attachment sites that develop as accessory ossification centers and mimic the maturation of an epiphyseal plate [1,24]. The calcaneal apophysis serves as the attachment site for the Achilles tendon superiorly and the plantar fascia inferiorly [16]. Inflammation of the calcaneal apophysis, known as Sever's disease, is one of the most common overuse injuries seen in the young athletic population, accounting for approximately 8% of all overuse injuries in this group [1,86]. It has been referred to as the ankle equivalent of Osgood-Schlatter's disease of the knee [16]. The typical presentation is that of an athlete who has just begun the season or has increased running activity recently. Pain is at the heel, particularly with running and jumping. Physical examination is often positive for tight Achilles' heel cord and weakness of the ankle dorsiflexors [1,87]. There also may be swelling and induration over the calcaneal apophysis. Diagnosis is usually clinical, and radiographs are usually not helpful. Treatment is multifaceted. First, causative activity should cease. Short-term icing and nonsteroidal anti-inflammatory drugs can be helpful for controlling the pain. A comprehensive program of heel cord stretching and dorsiflexor strengthening should be initiated. Barefoot walking should be avoided

because this prolonged traction is what leads to apophysitis. Occasionally, a heel insert or a heel lift is recommended to remove tensile forces on the tendon while the inflammation decreases [24,87].

Plantar fasciitis. The plantar fascia stretches from the calcaneal tuberosity and fans out to attach around the plantar aspect of the proximal phalanges [1]. Current literature has noted that this is not a true inflammatory condition but rather the result of repetitive microtrauma from continued athletic activity overuse [1,88,89]. Much like lateral epicondylitis, it seems that plantar fasciitis is not an "-itis" but rather an "-osis," a loss of normal tendon integrity. Young athletes involved with speed work, jumping, or hill running are at increased risk of developing this condition [16]. In young athletes, plantar fasciitis usually coincides with calcaneal apophysitis, but in adolescent athletes with closed physes, it can exist by itself and presents as medial arch or heel pain. Patients give a history of heavy athletic involvement and medial arch or heel pain, particularly with the first step out of bed every day. Physical examination shows tenderness over the anteromedial aspect of the heel, particularly with the foot in dorsiflexion [1]. This, like Sever's disease, is a clinical diagnosis, because radiographs are often not helpful. Treatment involves conservative measures, including relative rest, ice massage, arch supports, heel pads, and heel cord stretching and strengthening, both of which are paramount to successful rehabilitation. The decision to inject corticosteroids in the area is currently controversial in the literature, particularly in adolescent athletes. Evidence exists to support injection in adults, but complications such as tendon rupture and fat pad atrophy are real and must be monitored. Studies are not solid in adolescents [16].

Midfoot

Growth-related problems
Calcaneonavicular coalition. The two most common coalitions are the talocalcaneal and the calcaneonavicular coalitions. The calcaneonavicular coalition is a bony fusion between the talus and the calcaneus, and it is the second most common coalition behind the talocalcaneal coalition (Fig. 4). It has a similar presentation as the talocalcaneal coalition, with decreased range of motion across the hindfoot and the three-joint complex. Diagnosis and treatment are also similar.

Accessory navicular. An accessory navicular bone is the most common accessory bone in the foot [16]. It is an ossicle that develops like all other ossicles as a separate extrachondral ossification center, and it is located at the site of the tibialis posterior tendon insertion [14,16,90]. When it fails to ossify fully, it becomes an accessory navicular bone. It has been reported to occur in anywhere from 4% to 14% of the population [16]. It is not until adolescence, when athletes increase their participation, that these conditions

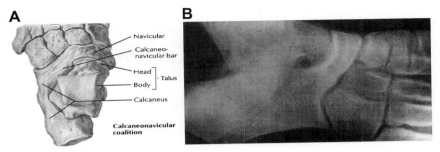

Fig. 4. (*A*) Pictorial of calcaneonavicular coalition. (*B*) Oblique radiograph shows the calcaneo-navicular fusion. (*Reprinted with permission from* Netter Anatomy Illustration Collection, © Elsevier Inc. All rights reserved.)

actually become painful. Patients present with pain medially along the arch of the foot, and on physical examination there is often a prominence along the arch of the foot that is tender with shoe wear [14]. Also on examination there is often evidence of pes planus. One theory about the development of pes planus is that the tibialis posterior tendon, which is a dynamic stabilizer of the medial longitudinal arch of the foot, inserts onto the accessory navicular instead of into the native navicular. Because it is a weaker insertion point, there is a drop in the longitudinal arch, which causes the pes planus [16]. Radiographic imaging is often diagnostic, but in cases in which it is not, MRI can help elucidate the lesion and define the anatomic points of insertion of the tibialis posterior tendon [72,91]. Treatment involves conservative management initially, with orthotics and casting and doughnut cut-outs for the painful parts over the enlarged navicular. If these measures fail and an athlete continues to have pain, there are well documented surgical procedures for the excision of these ossicles with varying degrees of handling of the posterior tibial tendon [14,92].

Overuse injuries
Navicular stress fractures. Aside from the previous discussion on stress fractures in general, one stress fracture in particular must be emphasized: the navicular stress fracture, which has been documented to have an incidence anywhere from 0% to 29% in young track and field athletes [15,93]. Navicular stress fractures are difficult to diagnose. The presentation is usually vague onset of foot pain along the dorsomedial area [10]. History elicits risk factors such as overuse with an increase in exercise duration and intensity and poor nutrition. Examination reveals palpatory tenderness over the dorsomedial navicular and may show mechanical configurations that may increase the risk of these fractures, such as a tight gastrocnemius complex or a Morton foot with a long second ray [10]. As with all stress fractures, radiographs are frequently normal, and a bone scan is required for definitive diagnosis. There must be a high incidence of suspicion for these fractures

because the navicular has poor blood supply over the middle one third, and if the fracture is untreated, poor healing with delayed union or nonunion is a possibility [10]. Treatment is more aggressive than with other stress fractures. Non–weight-bearing cast immobilization for 6 weeks is recommended by most physicians to prevent malunion, and if no progress is made, then surgical internal fixation is recommended. The usual time to return to athletic activity can be as long as 5 to 6 months [15,94].

Kohler's osteochondrosis. Osteochondroses are overuse lesions of the osteochondral ossification centers that are idiopathic. Osteochondrosis of the tarsal navicular is termed Kohler's disease. It typically occurs in children aged 5 to 9 years, and patients present with pain over the midfoot region that worsens with weight bearing [1]. Swelling of the area also may be present. Bilateral lesions have been known to occur, and one such case of bilateral lesions in twins led those authors to speculate on the possibility of a genetic predisposition to its occurrence [95]. Radiographs may be difficult to interpret because many children have irregular-appearing navicular bones that are normal and asymptomatic [1], but because patients have such good outcomes, further imaging has little use and does not change management. Treatment is conservative, with the use of the RICE technique and shoe supports for mild cases. Casting may be necessary over a 4- to 8-week period for more severe cases [95]. Patients typically fare well with this conservative treatment. In one series in the literature, 100% of patients became asymptomatic after conservative treatment, and the navicular returned to its normal appearance on radiographs [96]. There have been a few reports of children with Kohler's abnormality persisting into adulthood clinically and radiographically [97].

Acute injuries
Lisfranc injury. Lisfranc's joint is the tarsometatarsal articulation of the three cuneiforms and cuboid with the proximal five metatarsals. The keystones of this joint are the first and second metatarsals articulating with the first and second cuneiforms. Transverse ligaments connect the bases of the lateral four metatarsals; however, no such transverse ligament exists between the base of the first and second metatarsals. The second metatarsal proximally has small articulations with the three cuneiforms that support the tarsometatarsal articulation [1,98]. This is a precarious yet highly important anatomic location. Injuries at Lisfranc's joint can be in the form of sprains of the transverse ligaments or even fracture-dislocations. The most common mechanism of injury is an axial loading through the foot as the foot is forcefully plantarflexed and slightly rotated, which causes the proximal second metatarsal to dislocate dorsally [1,98,99]. Given this mechanism, many of the Lisfranc joint injuries seen in adolescents occur while playing football, with a large percentage of those injuries occurring in

linemen [1,100]. Linemen are often in situations in which other linemen step on their toes, which cause a heavy axial load while they are attempting to explode forward onto their toes.

The typical presentation involves an athlete with pain over the dorsum of the midfoot associated with swelling and an inability to bear weight through the midfoot, particularly on the tiptoes [1]. Plantar bruising often is associated with this injury, and if this sign is noticed, clinical suspicion should be raised. Radiographs are needed to make the diagnosis, particularly weight-bearing films (Fig. 5). There is a significantly high incidence of missed diagnoses [101]. One should look for malalignment between the first metatarsal and the first cuneiform or between the second metatarsal and the second cuneiform [99,101]. Severity grading is like other sprains, based on ligamentous tearing and amount of dislocation. Bone scans may help make the diagnosis in patients with negative radiographic results and continued high suspicion. Treatment of these injuries is based on the degree of severity. Stretch injuries or partial tears with less than 2 mm of malalignment should be treated conservatively with cast immobilization or a walking boot for 4 to 6 weeks [1,100]. Sprains that are more severe require operative reduction with internal fixation [1,102].

Forefoot

Overuse injuries
Iselin's apophysitis. Iselin's disease is an apophysitis that occurs at the tuberosity of the fifth metatarsal. The apophysis at this site appears at ages 9 to 14 and is located within the insertion of the peroneus brevis tendon

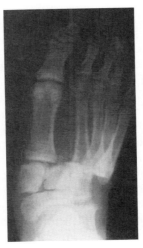

Fig. 5. Lisfranc injury. Note the malalignment between the metatarsals and the cuneiforms. (*Reprinted with permission from* Netter Anatomy Illustration Collection, © Elsevier Inc. All rights reserved.)

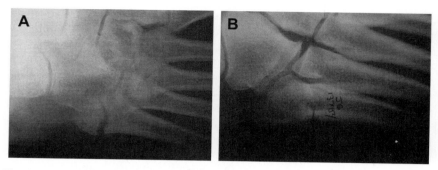

Fig. 6. (*A*) Fifth metatarsal avulsion fracture. (*B*) Jones fracture. Note how it extends to the metaphyseal-diaphyseal junction. (*Adapted from* Brodsky JW, Krause JO. Stress fractures of the foot and ankle. In: DeLee JC, Drez D, Miller MD, editors. Orthopaedic sports medicine: principles and practice. 2nd edition. Philadelphia: Saunders Elsevier; 2003. p. 2391–409; with permission.)

[16]. Presentation is similar to other cases of apophysitis in terms of history of overuse in athletically active older children. There is usually a presentation of insidious onset of pain over the lateral foot, with no history of trauma, in the setting of overuse-type activities. Radiographically, the apophysis appears as a diagonal or longitudinal line parallel to the long axis of the shaft of the fifth metatarsal, an important distinction from acute fifth metatarsal avulsion fractures, which are usually transverse in nature (see later discussion) [16]. Treatment is conservative, with decrease of activity and stretching and strengthening of the peroneal muscles. This treatment is usually effective until bony union eventually occurs [16].

Acute injuries
Fifth metatarsal fractures. Young child and adolescent athletes who present with pain along the lateral aspect of the foot near the fifth metatarsal present a challenging dilemma. History should be able to differentiate whether an acute or overuse injury has occurred; however, matters are not always that clear-cut. Three possible types of fractures are seen in the area of the base of the fifth metatarsal: include fifth metatarsal stress fractures, fifth metatarsal acute avulsion fractures, and Jones fractures. Metatarsal stress fractures are overuse injuries, which are the most common types of stress fractures seen in adolescent feet and ankles. Their management was reviewed previously. Most young athletes return to their sport in 4 to 6 weeks [16].

The fifth metatarsal acute fracture is the most common metatarsal fracture in children, accounting for 45% of all metatarsal fractures [16]. It occurs after an inversion-type injury, when the peroneus brevis tendon is avulsed from its attachment at the base of the fifth metatarsal [14]. Radiographs show the lesion, which can be distinguished from apophysitis because the fracture is transverse along the bone, whereas apophysitis of the fifth metatarsal (Iselin's

Table 1
Summary of common injuries of the foot and ankle in the child and adolescent athlete

	Lateral ankle	Medial & anterior ankle	Hindfoot	Midfoot	Forefoot
Growth problems		Medial malleolus ossification center	Talocalcaneal coalition Os trigonum	Calcaneonavicular coalition Accessory navicular	
Overuse injuries		Anterior ankle impingement syndrome	Sever's apophysitis Plantar fasciitis	Navicular stress fracture Kohler's apophysitis	Metatarsal stress fractures Iselin's disease
Acute injuries	Salter-Harris fractures Lateral ankle sprains Osteochondritis dissecans	Tillaux fractures Triplane fractures		Lisfranc injury	Fifth metatarsal avulsion fracture Jones fracture

disease) occurs along the diagonal plane from the bone (Fig. 6A) [16]. Treatment is usually conservative unless there is more than 2 to 3 mm of displacement, in which case surgical open reduction and internal fixation should be performed [14].

The Jones fracture is actually a fracture that occurs at the metaphyseal-diaphyseal junction of the base of the fifth metatarsal. The average age and demographics of occurrence of this fracture involve 15- to 21-year-old athletes [16]. Patients usually present with pain along the fifth metatarsal, particularly upon weight bearing, and give a history of an acute injury. Radiographs usually reveal the fracture (Fig. 6B). Similar to the navicular stress fracture, this lesion has higher rates of nonunion because it has poor blood supply to that area. Treatment involves a non–weight-bearing cast for 6 to 8 weeks and possible surgical screw fixation for nonhealing fractures [16].

Summary

Myriad problems in the foot and ankle are specific to child and adolescent athletes. The anatomy of young athletes with respect to the presence of a growth plate makes their injury patterns different from those seen in adults. The main general injury patterns seen in the feet and ankles of children are related to growth and development or occur from overuse syndromes or acute trauma. We have outlined in an anatomically oriented manner most of the common problems in this population. They are also summarized in Table 1.

References

[1] Pommering TL, Kluchurorski L, Hall SL. Ankle and foot injuries in pediatric and adult athletes. Prim Care 2005;32(1):133–61.

[2] Mahaffey D, Hilts M, Fields KB. Ankle and foot injuries in sports. Clinics in Family Practice 1999;1(1):233–50.

[3] Frey C, Bell J, Teresi L, et al. A comparison of MRI and clinical examination of acute lateral ankle sprains. Foot Ankle Int 1996;17(9):533–7.

[4] Damore DT, Metzl JD, Ramundo M, et al. Patterns in childhood sports injury. Pediatr Emerg Care 2003;19(2):65–7.

[5] Ruda SC. Common ankle injuries in the athlete. Nurs Clin North Am 1991;26(1):167–80.

[6] Garrick JB. The frequency of injury, mechanism of injury, and epidemiology of ankle sprains. Am J Sports Med 1977;5(6):242–50.

[7] Barr KP, Harrast MA. Evidence-based treatment of foot and ankle injuries in runners. Phys Med Rehabil Clin N Am 2005;16:779–99.

[8] Epperly T, Fields KB. Epidemiology of running injuries. In: O'Connor FG, Wilder RP, Nirschl R, editors. Textbook of running medicine. New York: McGraw-Hill; 2001. p. 3–9.

[9] Taunton JE, Ryan MB, Clement DB, et al. A retrospective case-control analysis of 2002 running injuries. Br J Sports Med 2002;36(2):95–101.

[10] Kennedy JG, Knowles B, Dolan M, et al. Foot and ankle injuries in the adolescent runner. Curr Opin Pediatr 2005;17(1):34–42.

[11] Kadel NJ. Foot and ankle injuries in dance. Phys Med Rehabil Clin N Am 2006;17:813–26.

[12] Chilvers M, Donahue M, Nassar L, et al. Foot and ankle injuries in elite female gymnasts. Foot Ankle Int 2007;28(2):214–8.

[13] Wojtys EM. Sports injuries in the immature athlete. Orthop Clin North Am 1987;18(4): 689–708.

[14] Chambers HG. Ankle and foot disorders in skeletally immature athletes. Orthop Clin North Am 2003;34(3):445–59.

[15] Pontell D, Hallivis R, Dollard MD. Sports injuries in the pediatric and adolescent foot and ankle: common overuse and acute presentations. Clin Podiatr Med Surg 2006;23(1):209–31.

[16] Omney ML, Micheli LJ. Foot and ankle problems in the young athlete. Med Sci Sports Exerc 1999;31(Suppl 7):S470–86.

[17] Elkus RA. Tarsal coalition in the young athlete. Am J Sports Med 1986;14(6):477–80.

[18] O'Neill DB, Micheli LJ. Tarsal coalition: a follow-up of adolescent athletes. Am J Sports Med 1989;17:544–9.

[19] MacGregor J. The skeletal system. In: MacGregor J, editor. Introduction to the anatomy and physiology of children. London: Routledge; 2000. p. 17–34.

[20] Hogan KA, Gross RH. Overuse injuries in pediatric athletes. Orthop Clin North Am 2003; 34(3):405–15.

[21] Herring SA, Nilson KL. Introduction to overuse injuries. Clin Sports Med 1987;6(2): 225–39.

[22] Stanitski CL. Overuse injuries. In: Stanitski CL, DeLee JC, Drez D, editors. Pediatric and adolescent sports medicine, vol 3. Philadelphia: WB Saunders Company; 1994. p. 94–9.

[23] Micheli LJ. Overuse injuries in children's sports: the growth factor. Orthop Clin North Am 1983;14(2):337–60.

[24] Carr KE. Musculoskeletal injuries in young athletes. Clin Fam Pract 2003;5(2):385–406.

[25] Resnick DR. Osteochondroses. In: Resnick DR, editor. Diagnosis of bone and joint disorders. 4th edition. Philadelphia: WB Saunders Company; 2002. p. 3686–741.

[26] Farmer JM, Martin DF, Boles CA, et al. Chondral and osteochondral injuries: diagnosis and management. Clin Sports Med 2001;20(2):299–320.

[27] Hershman EB, Mailly T. Stress fractures. Clin Sports Med 1990;9(1):183–214.

[28] Monteleone GP. Stress fractures in the athlete. Orthop Clin North Am 1995;26(3):423–32.

[29] Coady CM, Micheli LJ. Stress fractures in the pediatric athlete. Clin Sports Med 1997; 16(2):225–38.

[30] Beck BR, Matheson GO. Common stress fractures. Clin Fam Pract 1999;1(1):251–74.

[31] Orava S, Jromakka E, Hulkko A. Stress fractures in young athletes. Arch Orthop Trauma Surg 1981;98:271.

[32] Verma RB, Sherman O. Athletic stress fractures. Part I: history, epidemiology, physiology, risk factors, radiology, diagnosis and treatment. Am J Orthop 2001;30(11):798–806.

[33] Milgrom C, Finestone A, Shlamkovitch N, et al. Youth as a risk factor for stress fracture: a study of 783 infantry recruits. J Bone Joint Surg 1994;76-B(1):20–2.

[34] Frusztajer NT, Dhuper S, Warren MP, et al. Nutrition and the incidence of stress fractures in ballet dancers. Am J Clin Nutr 1990;51(5):779–83.

[35] Giladi M, Milgorm C, Simkin A, et al. Stress fractures: identifiable risk factors. Am J Sports Med 1991;19(6):647–52.

[36] Margulies JY, Simkin A, Leichter I, et al. Effect of intense physical activity on the bone-mineral content in the lower limbs of young adults. J Bone Joint Surg Am 1986;68(7): 1090–3.

[37] Stanitski C. Management of sports injuries in children and adolescents. Orthop Clin North Am 1998;19:689–98.

[38] Rettig AC, Shelbourne KD, Beltz HF, et al. Radiographic evaluation of foot and ankle injuries in the athlete. Clin Sports Med 1987;6(4):905–19.

[39] Matheson GO, Clement DB, McKenzie DC, et al. Stress fractures in athletes: a study of 320 cases. Am J Sports Med 1987;15(1):46–58.

[40] Gross RH. Foot and ankle injuries and disorders. Adolescent Medicine State of the Art Reviews 1998;9(3):599–609.

[41] Ashhurst APC, Bromer RS. Classification and mechanism of fractures of the leg bones involving the ankle. Arch Surg 1922;4:121–9.

[42] Dias LS, Giegerich CR. Fractures of the distal tibial epiphysis in adolescence. J Bone Joint Surg 1983;65(4):438–44.

[43] Dias L, Tachdjian M. Physical injuries of the ankle in children. Clin Orthop 1978;136: 230–3.

[44] Landin L, Danielsson L. Children's ankle fractures. Acta Orthop Scand 1983;54:634–40.

[45] Lauge-Hansen N. Fractures of the ankle. II: combined experimental surgical and experimental roentgenologic investigations. Arch Surg 1950;60:957.

[46] Salter R, Harris W. Injuries involving the epiphyseal plate. J Bone Joint Surg 1963;45: 587–622.

[47] Brown JH, DeLuca SA. Growth plate injuries: Salter-Harris classification. Am Fam Physician 1992;46(4):1180–4.

[48] Devalentine SJ. Epiphyseal injuries of the foot and ankle. Clin Podiatr Med Surg 1987;4(1): 279–310.

[49] Goldberg VM, Aadalen R. Distal tibial epiphyseal injuries: the role of athletics in 53 cases. Am J Sports Med 1978;6(5):263–8.

[50] Pizzutillo PD, Chandler JB, Maxwell T. Pediatric orthopedics: fractures of the growth plate. In: Griffin LY, editor. Essentials of musculoskeletal care. 3rd edition. Rosemont (IL): American Academy of Orthopedic Surgeons; 2005. Section 9. p. 865–7.

[51] Rohmiller MT, Gaynor TP, Pawelek J, et al. Salter-Harris I and II fractures of the distal tibia: does mechanism of injury relate to premature physeal closure? J Pediatr Orthop 2006;26(3):322–8.

[52] Norkin CC, Levangie PK. The ankle-foot complex. In: Norkin CC, Levangie PK, editors. Joint structure and function: a comprehensive analysis. Philadelphia: FA Davis Company; 1992. p. 379–418.

[53] Kitaoka HB, Crevoisier XM, Hansen D, et al. Foot and ankle kinematics and ground reaction forces during ambulation. Foot Ankle Int 2006;27(10):808–13.

[54] Bennett WF. Lateral ankle sprains. Part I: anatomy, biomechanics, diagnosis, and natural history. Orthop Rev 1994;23(5):381–7.

[55] Cohen RS, Balcom TA. Current treatment options for ankle injuries: lateral ankle sprain, Achilles tendonitis, and Achilles rupture. Curr Sports Med Rep 2003;2(5):251–4.

[56] Young CC, Niedfeldt MW, Morris GA, et al. Clinical examination of the foot and ankle. Primary Care: Clinics in Office Practice 2005;32(1):105–32.

[57] Hyman GS, Solomon J, Dahm D. Physical examination of the foot and ankle. In: Malanga GA, Nadler SF, editors. Musculoskeletal physical examination: an evidence-based approach. Philadelphia: Elsevier Mosby; 2006. p. 315–43.

[58] Brown DP, Freeman ED, Cuccurullo SJ. Musculoskeletal medicine. In: Cuccurullo SJ, editor. Physical medicine and rehabilitation board review. New York: Demos; 2004. p. 131–293.

[59] Clark KD, Tanner S. Evaluation of the Ottawa ankle rules in children. Pediatr Emerg Care 2003;19(2):73–8.

[60] Stiell IG, Greenberg GH, McKnight RD, et al. A study to develop clinical decision rules for the use of radiography in acute ankle injuries. Ann Emerg Med 1992;21(4):384–90.

[61] Churchill JA, Mazur JM. Ankle pain in children: diagnostic evaluation and clinical decision making. J Am Acad Orthop Surg 1995;3(4):183–93.

[62] Boutis K, Komar L, Jaramillo D, et al. Sensitivity of a clinical examination to predict need for radiography in children with ankle injuries: a prospective study. Lancet 2001;358(9299): 2118–21.

[63] Smith RW, Reischl SF. Treatment of ankle sprains in young athletes. Am J Sports Med 1986;14(6):465–71.

[64] Bennett WF. Lateral ankle sprains. Part II: acute and chronic treatment. Orhtop Rev 1994; 23(6):504–10.

[65] Safran MR, Zachazewski JE, Benedetti RS, et al. Lateral ankle sprains: a comprehensive review. Part 2: treatment and rehabilitation with an emphasis on the athlete. Med Sci Sports Exerc 1999;31(7):S438–47.

[66] Stonnington MJ. Lower leg, ankle and foot. In: Buschbacher RS, editor. Practical guide to musculoskeletal disorders: diagnosis and rehabilitation. 2nd edition. Boston: Butterworth Heinemann; 2002. p. 229–54.

[67] Mascaro TB, Swanson LE. Rehabilitation of the foot and ankle. Orthop Clin North Am 1994;25(1):147–60.

[68] Safran MR, Benedtti RS, Bartolzzi AR, et al. Lateral ankle sprains: a comprehensive review part 1: etiology, pathoanatomy, histopathogenesis and diagnosis. Med Sci Sports Exerc 1999;31(7):S429–37.

[69] Sullivan JA. Ankle and foot injuries in the pediatric athlete. Instr Course Lect 1993;42: 545–51.

[70] Pizzutillo P. The osteochondroses. In: Sullivan JA, Grana WA, editors. The pediatric athlete. Park Ridge (IL): American Academy of Orthopaedic Surgeons; 1990. p. 211–33.

[71] Canale ST, Belding RH. Osteochondral lesions of the talus. J Bone Joint Surg 1980;62(4): 97–102.

[72] Canale ST. Osteochondroses and related problems of the foot and ankle. In: DeLee JC, Drez D, Miller MD, editors. Orthopedic sports medicine: principles and practice. 2nd edition. Philadelphia: Saunders; 2003. p. 2587–623.

[73] Brendt AL, Harty M. Transchondral fractures (osteochondritis dissecans) of the talus. J Bone Joint Surg 1959;41(4):988–1020.

[74] Smith DK, Gilley JS. Imaging of sports injuries of the foot and ankle. In: DeLee JC, Drez D, Miller MD, editors. Orthopedic sports medicine: principles and practice. 2nd edition. Philadelphia: Saunders; 2003. p. 2190–224.

[75] Sullivan JA. Ligament injuries of the foot/ankle in the pediatric athlete. In: DeLee JC, Drez D, Miller MD, editors. Orthopedic sports medicine: principles and practice. 2nd edition. Philadelphia: Saunders; 2003. p. 2376–91.

[76] Stanitski CL, Micheli LJ. Observations on symptomatic medial malleolar ossification centers. J Pediatr Orthop 1993;13(2):164–8.

[77] Hunter-Griffin LY. Injuries to the leg, ankle and foot. In: Sullivan JA, Granna WA, editors. The pediatric athlete. Park Ridge (IL): American Academy of Orthopaedic Surgeons; 1990. p. 187–98.

[78] Cooperman D, Spiegel P, Laros G. Tibial fractures involving the ankle in children. J Bone Joint Surg 1978;60(8):1040–6.

[79] Lynn M. The triplane distal epiphyseal fracture. Clin Orthop 1972;86:187–90.

[80] Cone R, Nygayen V, Fluornoy J, et al. Triplane fracture of the distal tibial epiphysis. Radiology 1984;153(3):763–7.

[81] Bohne WHO. Tarsal coalition. Curr Opin Pediatr 2001;13(1):29–35.

[82] Cowell HR. Talocalcaneal coalition and new causes of peroneal spastic flatfoot. Clin Orthop 1972;85:16–22.

[83] Harty MP. Imaging of pediatric foot disorders. Radiol Clin North Am 2001;39(4):733–48.

[84] Marotta JJ, Micheli LJ. Os trigonum impingement in dancers. Am J Sports med 1992;20(5): 533–6.

[85] Quirk R. Talar compression syndrome in dancers. Foot Ankle 1982;3(2):65–8.

[86] Maffulli N, Wong J, Almekinders LC. Types and epidemiology of tendinopathy. Clin Sports Med 2003;22(4):675–92.

[87] Christopher NC, Cogeni J. Overuse injuries in the pediatric athlete: evaluation, initial management, and strategies for prevention. Clinical Pediatric Emergency Medicine 2002; 3(2):118–28.

[88] Lemont H, Ammirati KM, Usen N. Plantar fasciitis: a degenerative process (fasciosis) without inflammation. J Am Podiatr Med Assoc 2003;93(3):234–7.

[89] Wapner KL, Bordelon RL. Heel pain. In: DeLee JC, Drez D, Miller MD, editors. Orthopedic sports medicine: principles and practice. 2nd edition. Philadelphia: Saunders; 2003. p. 2446–72.

[90] Grogan DP, Gasser SI, Ogden JA. The painful accessory navicular: a clinical and histopathological study. Foot Ankle 1989;10(3):164–9.

[91] Kitter E, Edrag N, Karatosun V, et al. Tibialis posterior tendon abnormalities in feet with accessory navicular bone and flat foot. Acta Orthop Scand 1999;70:618–21.

[92] Ugolini PA, Raikin SM. The accessory navicular. Foot Ankle Clin 2004;9(1):165–80.

[93] Bennell KL, Brukner PD. Epidemiology and site specificity of stress fractures. Clin Sports Med 1997;16(2):179–96.

[94] Khan KM, Fuller PJ, Brukner PD. Outcome of conservative and surgical management of navicular stress fracture and athletes. Am J Sports Med 1992;20(6):657–66.

[95] Tsirikos AI, Riddle EC, Kruse R. Bilateral Kohler's disease in identical twins. Clin Orthop Relat Res 2003;409:195–8.

[96] Williams GA, Cowell HR. Kohler's disease of the tarsal navicular. Clin Orthop 1981;158: 53–8.

[97] Sharp RJ, Calder JD, Saxby TS. Osteochondrosis of the navicular: a case report. Foot Ankle Int 2003;24(6):509–13.

[98] Kay MR, Tang CW. Pediatric foot fractures: evaluation and treatment. J Am Acad Orthop Surg 2001;9(5):308–19.

[99] Kolodin EL, Vitale T. Foot disorders. In: DeLisa JA, editor. Physical medicine and rehabilitation: principles and practice and practice. 4th edition. Philadelphia: Lipincott Williams and Wilkins; 2005. p. 873–94.

[100] Nunley JA, Vertullo CJ. Classification, investigation and management of midfoot sprains. Am J Sports Med 2002;30(6):871–8.

[101] Sherief TI, Mucci B, Greiss M. Lisfranc injury: how frequently does it get missed? And how can we improve? Injury 2007;38(7):856–60.

[102] Philbin T, Rosenberg G, Sferra JJ. Complications of missed or untreated Lisfranc injuries. Foot Ankle Clin N Am 2003;8(1):61–71.

ELSEVIER
SAUNDERS

Phys Med Rehabil Clin N Am
19 (2008) 373–398

PHYSICAL MEDICINE
AND REHABILITATION
CLINICS OF
NORTH AMERICA

Nutritional Requirements of the Child and Teenage Athlete

Anne Z. Hoch, DO, MD, PT*,
Katie Goossen, BS, Tricia Kretschmer, BS

*Department of Orthopaedic Surgery, Medical College of Wisconsin,
9200 W Wisconsin Avenue, Milwaukee, WI 53226, USA*

There has been an explosion in sports participation, especially for women, in the last 35 years mainly because of Title IX. In 2005–2006, nearly 3 million girls and 4.2 million boys participated in high school athletics, and many more participated in club sports and recreational activities. On the other end of the spectrum, the prevalence of obesity in the United States is at an all-time high. Proper nutrition in combination with the appropriate amount of physical activity is of paramount importance for this era of adolescents.

Growth

Boys and girls typically follow specific patterns of growth from infancy to adulthood. Infancy and early childhood are characterized by a period of rapid growth. Middle childhood is typically a period of small, constant gains. Adolescence is again characterized by rapid growth, and then growth is relatively slow and constant until adulthood. School-aged children and adolescents are at a critical time period because nutritional deficiencies could have a significant effect not only on growth and development but also on athletic and academic performance. Before puberty, there is no significant difference between boys and girls in regards to biomechanics, body composition, or nutritional requirements.

It is challenging to make general recommendations for nutritional needs for adolescents because not only age but also stage of physical maturity and

* Corresponding author.
E-mail address: azeni@mcw.edu (A.Z. Hoch).

level of physical activity must be considered. The dietary reference intakes, which include the recommended dietary allowances (RDA), adequate intakes (AI), and tolerable upper intakes levels for adolescents, are stated for three age groups, as shown in Table 1.

Caloric needs for adolescents vary considerably depending on age, growth rate, and level of physical maturity. The RDA for caloric and protein needs for male and female individuals aged 11 to 24 are shown in Table 2. Calories per unit height (cm) and weight (kg) can be used for general estimates. However, this does not reflect energy expenditure from exercise or growth rate.

The role of carbohydrates, proteins, and fats in athletic performance

Basic nutrition is vital for aiding in growth, providing energy, and achieving good health and school performance. Sports nutrition expands on these basic principles to enhance athletic performance by reducing fatigue and susceptibility to disease and injury while concurrently allowing an athlete to train harder and longer and recover faster [1]. The underlying macronutrients that fuel physical activity are carbohydrates, proteins, and fats. It is crucial for athletes to take in equal or more calories than they are expending to prevent an energy deficit, which can result in loss of muscle mass, menstrual dysfunction, loss of or failure to gain bone density, and increased risk for fatigue, injury, or illness [2].

In order for any muscle to do work, adenosine triphosphate (ATP) is required; it also must be replenished continuously during physical activity in order for the activity to continue [3]. When energy demands increase during exercise, the body relies on three different systems to transfer stored energy to ATP: the phosphagen, glycolytic, and aerobic systems [3]. The phosphagen system uses stored phosphocreatine in muscle cells to directly produce ATP and is used primarily for short-term, high-intensity exercise, such as sprinting, high jumping, or a rapid weight lift. Myocytes can only store small amounts of phosphocreatine, however, and ATP production is limited accordingly. This system can only deliver enough ATP to support activity that lasts less than 20 seconds. The glycolytic system is also a short-term fuel provider and supplies ATP for intense activity that lasts from 20 to 45 seconds [4]. Both of these systems are anaerobic, whereas the third system, oxidative phosphorylation, requires oxygen to produce ATP through the oxidation of carbohydrates, fats, and proteins. This system is used for activity lasting longer than 45 seconds [4].

In 2005, the government introduced a revision of their food guidance system. Originally, it was developed in 1992 as the food pyramid guide (FPG). "MyPyramid," released in 2005, symbolizes a personalized approach to healthy eating and physical activity (Figs. 1 and 2). It is recommended for everyone to obtain at least the lower end of the recommended range of servings, whereas the higher end is suggested for athletes who expend a significant amount of energy in physical activity. The Institutes of

Table 1
Food and Nutrition Board, National Academy of Sciences—National Research Council recommended dietary allowances, revised 1989 (abridged)

	Age (y)	Weight[a] (kg)	Weight[a] (lb)	Height[a] (cm)	Height[a] (in)	Vitamin A (µg RE)[b]	Vitamin D (µg)[c]	Vitamin E (mg α-TE)[d]	Vitamin K (µg)	Vitamin C (mg)	Iron (mg)	Zinc (mg)	Iodine (µg)	Selenium (µg)
Children	4–6	20	44	112	44	500	10	7	20	45	10	10	90	20
	7–10	28	62	132	52	700	10	7	30	45	10	10	120	30
Males	11–14	45	99	157	62	1000	10	10	45	50	12	15	150	40
	15–18	66	145	176	69	1000	10	10	65	60	12	15	150	50
	19–24	72	160	177	70	1000	10	10	70	60	10	15	150	70
	25–50	79	174	176	70	1000	5	10	80	60	10	15	150	70
Females	11–14	46	101	157	62	800	10	8	45	50	15	12	150	45
	15–18	55	120	163	64	800	10	8	55	60	15	12	150	50
	19–24	58	128	164	65	800	10	8	60	60	15	12	150	55
	25–50	63	138	163	64	800	5	8	65	60	15	12	150	55

The recommended dietary allowances are designed for the maintenance of good nutrition of practically all healthy people in the United States. This table does not include nutrients for which dietary reference intakes have recently been established [5,6]. The allowances, expressed as average daily intakes over time, are intended to provide for individual variations among most normal persons as they live in the United States under usual environmental stresses. Diets should be based on a variety of common foods to provide other nutrients for which human requirements have been less well defined.

[a] Weights and heights of reference adults are actual medians for the US population of the designated age, as reported by National Health and Nutrition Examination Survey II. The use of these figures does not imply that the height-to-weight ratios are ideal.

[b] Retinol equivalents: 1 retinol equivalent = 1 µg retinol or 6 µg β-carotene.

[c] As cholecalciferol: 10 µg cholecalciferol = 400 IU of vitamin D.

[d] α-Tocopherol equivalents: 1 mg d-α tocopherol = 1 α-TE. See text for variation in allowances and calculation of vitamin E activity of the diet as α-tocopherol equivalents.

From Recommended Dietary Allowances. 10th ed. © 1998 by the National Academy of Sciences. Washington, DC: National Academy Press; with permission.

Table 2
Recommended energy and protein allowances

	Age (y)	Weight		Height		Energy		Protein	
		(kg)	(lb)	(cm)	(in)	Kcal/d	Kcal/kg	g/d	g/kg[a]
Children	4–6	20	44	112	44	1800	90	24	1.1
	7–10	28	62	132	52	2000	70	28	1.0
Males	11–14	45	99	157	62	2500	55	45	1.0
	15–18	66	145	176	69	3000	45	59	0.9
	19–24	72	160	177	70	2900	40	58	0.8
	25–50	79	174	176	70	2900	37	63	0.8
Females	11–14	46	101	157	62	2200	47	46	1.0
	15–18	55	120	163	64	2200	40	44	0.8
	19–24	58	128	164	65	2200	38	46	0.8
	25–50	63	138	163	64	2200	36	80	0.8

[a] Amino acid score of typical United States diet is 100 for all age groups, except young infants. Digestibility is equal to reference proteins. Values have been rounded upward to 0.1 g/kg.

From Recommended Dietary Allowances. 10th ed. © 1998 by the National Academy of Sciences. Washington, DC: National Academy Press; with permission.

Medicine Food and Nutrition Board recently revised caloric recommendations as follows [3]:

Male athletes aged 30 years and older

Total energy expenditure $= 662 - 9.53 \times$ age (years) $+ 1.48$ [physical activity] $\times (15.91 \times$ weight [kg] $+ 539.6 \times$ height [m])

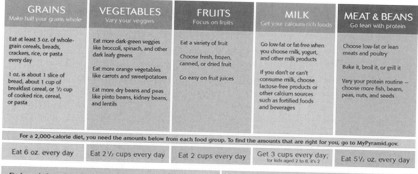

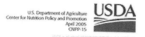

Fig. 1. U.S. Department of Agriculture dietary guidelines for adults. (*Courtesy of* the USDA Center for Nutrition Policy and Promotion, Alexandria, VA.)

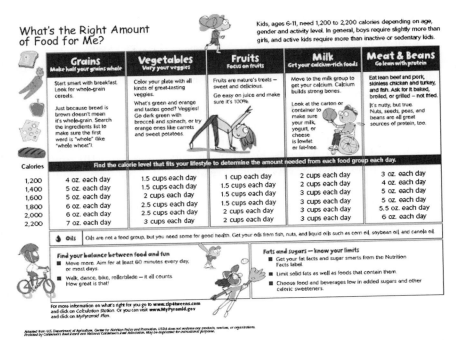

Fig. 2. U.S. Department of Agriculture dietary guidelines for children. (*Courtesy of* the USDA Center for Nutrition Policy and Promotion, Alexandria, VA.)

Female athletes aged 30 years and older

Total energy expenditure $= 354 - 6.91 \times$ age (years) $+ 1.45$ [physical activity] $\times (9.36 \times$ weight [kg] $+ 726 \times$ height [m])

For male and female athletes between 19 and 30 years

Add 7 kcal/d for women and 10 kcal/d for men for every year before 30

For children and teens younger than 19 years

Boys/girls aged 7 to 10: 2000 calories/d

High school boys: 3000 to 6000 calories/d

High school girls: 2200 to 4000 calories/d

Carbohydrates are the primary source of fuel during exercise and contain approximately 4 kcal/g. An adult athlete's diet should typically be made up of 60% to 65% carbohydrates, whereas an adolescent athlete's diet should contain 55% to 60% [7]. In 2002, the Institute of Medicine established the RDA of carbohydrates for adults and children as 130 g/d, which is based on the amount needed to supply the brain with adequate glucose [8]. Beyond this specific RDA, they also set for carbohydrates an acceptable macronutrient distribution range of 45% to 65% of total caloric intake. Both of these guidelines are intended to meet the needs of 95% of the general population [6].

Carbohydrates taken in through food are necessary to maintain blood glucose and is stored as glycogen in the muscles and liver [4]. Muscle glycogen is the fastest form of energy available to the working muscle and can be released up to three times quicker than energy from any other source [7]. Muscle glycogen and blood glucose are also the limiting factors in any type of human performance [8]. As exercise intensity increases, the more muscle glycogen is relied on as an energy source [9]; however, as the duration of exercise increases, the source of energy shifts from muscle glycogen to circulating blood glucose [2]. During long periods of exercise, muscle glycogen and blood glucose levels both become low, and unless carbohydrates are replenished, an athlete will not be able to perform at a high level [1,8,9]. A study by Ahlborg and colleagues [10] found that work time to exhaustion was directly related to the quantity of initial glycogen stores in the working muscles. They showed that by manipulating the quantity of carbohydrate in the diet, the concentration of glycogen in the muscle could be altered, as could the athlete's time to exhaustion.

Endurance athletes who train aerobically for more than 90 minutes daily need approximately 6 to 10 g of carbohydrate/kg of body weight/day to restore glycogen levels during training. This amounts to roughly 300 to 700 g of carbohydrate [1,2,8]. Carbohydrate ingestion during exercise that lasts longer than 1 hour also may help increase endurance [2,8,11]. Athletes can help maintain their body's supply of energy by consuming approximately 25 to 30 g of carbohydrate every half hour during exercise. This practice can improve performance by maintaining blood glucose levels after muscle glycogen has been diminished, because 1 g carbohydrate/min is delivered to the tissues as fatigue sets in [8].

Proteins carry out many bodily functions and aid in the structure of skin, hair, nails, and muscle. Protein normally provides less than 5% of the energy expended at rest and during mild exercise [12]. However, as exercise duration increases, proteins contribute to the maintenance of blood glucose via gluconeogenesis in the liver [2]. Proteins contain approximately 4 kcal/g, similar to carbohydrates, and the current RDA for protein is 0.8 g/kg body weight/day for the general population.

Athletes may require a higher protein intake in the early stages of resistance and endurance training because of increasing muscle mass [13]. In the beginning of training, the recommended protein intake is 1.5 to 1.7 g/kg body weight/day. As training enters the maintenance phase, protein intake may be decreased to 1.0 to 1.4 g/kg body weight/day. Protein requirements are necessarily greater in adolescents than in sedentary adults because of growth and development of lean body mass. The RDA of protein for active children and adolescents is 2 g/kg/d [5]. Overall, the protein recommendation for active adults and children is 12% to15% of energy intake [8,13]. Resistance training may require a higher protein intake, and weight lifters consume anywhere from 1.2 to 3.4 g/kg body weight/day [8]. Bodily protein synthesis seems to be at a maximum in strength-training athletes who consume 1.4 g protein/kg body weight/day [14].

Consuming more protein than the body can use is unnecessary and should be avoided. This is an important guideline to remember as ergogenic aids and other supplements become increasingly popular in modern society. When athletes consume diets that are high in protein, they compromise their carbohydrate status, which may affect their ability to train and compete at peak levels. Taking large amounts of protein or amino acid supplements can also lead to dehydration, urinary loss of calcium, weight gain, and stress on the kidneys and liver because protein requires almost seven times more water for metabolism than fat or carbohydrates [8,12].

Fats are used as a secondary fuel source after carbohydrates. Fats provide necessary vitamins, are essential for menstrual function, and protect the internal organs. They contain 9 kcal/g and should make up 20% to 25% of an athlete's diet. There is no specific RDA for fat intake, but it is recommended that athletes consume no more than is recommended for a sedentary person. Children and adults should take in no more than 10% saturated, 10% polyunsaturated, and 10% monounsaturated fats in their diet.

Fat is the major fuel for light- to moderate-intensity exercise ($<60\%$ VO_{2max}). During low-intensity exercise that lasts longer than 30 minutes, there is a gradual shift away from carbohydrate metabolism with an increasing reliance on fat metabolism, or beta-oxidation, as the primary energy source [4]. With training, the quantity of mitochondrial enzymes can increase, which in turn increases fatty acid oxidation. Glucose uptake, glycolysis, and glycogenolysis are then increasingly inhibited by free fatty acid oxidation within the skeletal muscle [13]. Trained individuals are able to use fat stores more efficiently than untrained athletes, who rely more heavily on carbohydrate stores.

One aspect of performance unique to women and younger adolescents is their higher capacity for lipid oxidation [1,5,15]. Women are believed to oxidize fat better than men because of fluctuating hormones in the menstrual cycle. These hormones dramatically influence substrate selection and most likely account for the reduced reliance on carbohydrates [16]. Children and adolescents generally have higher levels of glycerol in their blood, which results in increased use of free fatty acids during exercise. Despite their increased lipid use, it is still recommended that an adolescent's consumption of fats be no more than 30% of their daily caloric intake [5].

It is important for physically active children and adolescents to consume enough nutrients to meet their needs for growth, tissue maintenance, and physical and intellectual performance [5]. It is difficult to establish specific recommended intakes, however, because of large individual variability. During growth spurts, adolescents should consume an additional 500 kcal/d above their usual intake [17,18]. Carbohydrates do not seem to play as great a role for youth in exercise as for adults because of the submaximal glycolytic capacity characteristic of younger age [5,17,19]. The RDA for carbohydrates in children and adolescents is at least 50% of total daily caloric intake. The children's FPG (see Fig. 2) is a useful tool for ensuring adequate nutrition in the diet. It is important to remember that active children should consume the high end of the range of recommended servings for each food group.

Precompetition meals are essential for athletes to maintain energy levels for the exercising muscles during competition [8]. In a study by Sherman and colleagues, cycling performance was improved by 15% when athletes consumed 4.5 g/kg body weight carbohydrate 4 hours before moderate-intensity exercise. Consuming 1 to 4.5 g of carbohydrate/kg body weight 1 to 4 hours before activity helps to maintain blood glucose levels during exercise and ensure adequate carbohydrate availability [1,20]. It is not recommended for athletes to fast before competition because of the risk of their blood glucose levels decreasing during exercise and impairing performance [1].

A study by Thomas and colleagues [21] also showed that the glycemic index of an individual's food intake may affect performance. Cyclists who consumed low glycemic index carbohydrates (<60) 1 hour before pedaling to exhaustion had a significantly longer endurance time than individuals who consumed medium (60–80) and high glycemic foods (>80). High glycemic foods cause a rapid surge in blood glucose levels, which may then cause a quick release of insulin to counteract that rise. Low glycemic foods are optimal for supplying long-term sustained energy for children and adults without causing pendulous swings in blood sugar [1,5,21]. Examples of low glycemic index foods include whole grain products, low-fat yogurt or milk, apples, and almost all vegetables and beans [8]. The pre-event meal should be high in carbohydrate and low in fat so that it may be easily digested. Excess fat should not be consumed because it delays stomach emptying and takes longer to digest. Excess protein also should be avoided to prevent added stress on the kidneys. The meal should be eaten 3.5 to 4 hours before an event and provide 100 to 200 g carbohydrate for children and adolescents [8]. Appropriate pregame meals include toast with jelly, a baked potato, spaghetti with tomato sauce, cereal with skim milk, or low-fat yogurt with fruit [8]. Anyone who competes in all-day events should consume 1 g of carbohydrate/kg body weight for every hour of activity. Good sources include fresh fruits, energy bars, and sports drinks [8].

The 2 hours after competition represent the most critical time to restore muscle glycogen; synthesis is reduced by 66% when postexercise carbohydrate ingestion is delayed more than 2 hours [8]. Athletes should consume at least 1.5 g of carbohydrate/kg body weight immediately after exercise and again 2 hours after exercise to maximize glycogen regeneration. Carbohydrates with a medium to high glycemic index should take priority in postexercise recovery diets. Good sources of these foods include white bread, raisins, bananas, sugar, carrots, pasta, honey, and sports drinks [11,13]. A study by Burke and colleagues demonstrated that consuming high glycemic carbohydrate foods produced greater glycogen storage in the first 24 hours after exercise than did low glycemic index foods [1,2,22]. Increased protein intake is also recommended for muscle repair and to further increase the glycogen resynthesis rate. Good foods to consume that have both protein and carbohydrates include peanut butter or cheese with crackers, trail mix, sports bars, and yogurt and granola. Guidelines recommend a 1:3 ratio of protein to carbohydrate consumption [3].

Elite athletes, recreational athletes, and sedentary people all require the same nutrients, although the amount of nutrients needed is influenced by age, sex, body size, activity level, and state of health [1]. It is important for all athletes to consume a balanced diet that consists of approximately 50% to 65% carbohydrates, 20% to 30% fats, and 12% to 15% proteins to ensure health and performance. Proper nutrition in young athletes is vital to prevent inadequate energy intake, which may inhibit normal growth and development [5] and overall performance.

Calcium

Calcium is an essential mineral that is important for bone health and muscle contraction and normal enzyme activity. Approximately 1 kg of the 1.2 kg of calcium in the body is present in bones and teeth, but it is important to recognize that bone is constantly being deposited and resorbed, with the net process depending on how much calcium is taken in from the diet [23]. Calcium is lost through sweat, urine, and feces, so enough calcium must be consumed daily to compensate for these losses. Absorption of calcium in the gastrointestinal tract depends on the availability of active 1,25-dihydroxyvitamin D, which is in turn regulated by the parathyroid gland and parathyroid hormone (PTH) [23]. When the parathyroid gland senses low calcium in the extracellular fluid, PTH is released and causes (1) increased conversion of vitamin D to the active form (by the kidney), (2) increased absorption of calcium from the gut, and (3) increased resorption of bone to maintain plasma calcium at acceptable levels. Failure of this regulation can lead to hypocalcemia or hypercalcemia [23].

There is much debate about what constitutes a sufficient daily intake of calcium, especially for adolescents, but the recommendation set by the 1997 National Academy of Sciences is 1300 mg/d for 9- to 18-year-old individuals [26]. Instead of referring to this as the RDA, they instead use the term "adequate intake" (AI). National Academy of Sciences AI guidelines are intended to meet the dietary requirements of 95% of the population of healthy subjects [26]. Previously, the 1994 NIH Consensus Conference recommended 800 to 1200 mg of calcium per day for 6- to 10-year-old children and 1200 to 1500 mg/d for 11- to 18-year-old individuals [5]. The tolerable upper limit for calcium intake is 2500 mg/d for all age groups; above this, zinc and iron absorption may be affected [27].

Further research has investigated the differences between men and women with regard to calcium requirements during adolescence. Girls tend to reach puberty approximately 2 to 3 years earlier than boys and progress through the five Tanner stages of development at different ages than their male counterparts. Boys, however, tend to spend approximately 6 years in puberty as compared with girls' 4 years [28]. One study showed that girls retain almost four times as much calcium in Tanner stages I–III than during stages IV and V [29]. Although a similar study was not done in boys, these results indicate that calcium requirements likely change depending on the stage of adolescence. The role of vitamin D also should not be overlooked. A 2005 study of adults indicated that a serum 25-hydroxyvitamin D level of 18 ng/mL is sufficient to maintain ideal serum PTH, despite calcium intake of less than 800 mg/d [30]. When serum vitamin D levels are insufficient, even a daily calcium intake of more than 1200 mg is not enough to prevent increased serum PTH and increased bone resorption [30].

Calcium is present in a wide variety of foods and beverages, with milk, yogurt, and cheese contributing the most calcium to the typical American diet [31]. One 8-oz glass of milk, one cup of yogurt, and 1.5 oz of cheese each contains approximately 300 mg of calcium [27]. Certain vegetables, such as kale, broccoli, and spinach, and fortified juices and grain products can help people who avoid dairy products or are lactose intolerant still reach the recommended calcium intake, although on average these items contain significantly less calcium than dairy products. Soy milk, a popular alternative to regular milk, varies widely between brands and types, containing anywhere from 80 to 500 mg of calcium in an 8-oz glass [27]. A common misconception is that dairy products are all fattening and should be avoided by dieters; in fact, the opposite is true. One recent study showed that obtaining sufficient dietary calcium from dairy products actually accelerated weight and fat loss when combined with dieting compared with caloric restriction with minimal dairy intake and insufficient calcium [32].

An NIH news release in 2001 called attention to what is termed a "calcium crisis" affecting our youth. Of youth aged 12 to 19 years in the United States, only 13.5% of girls and 36.3% of boys get the recommended daily intake of calcium [33]. Bone mineral density normally increases during childhood and adolescence until approximately age 20, when peak bone mass is achieved [19]. Studies also have shown a correlation between peak bone mass attained during adolescence and future risk for the development of osteoporosis [34]. As such, the overwhelming negative calcium balance seen in youth is "a pediatric disease with geriatric consequences" [33].

Adolescent athletes are a group especially at risk for calcium deficiency because athletes often restrict their caloric intake by decreasing consumption of dairy products [2]. In 1997, the American College of Sports Medicine described an emerging pattern in women's athletics known as the female athlete triad, characterized by disordered eating, amenorrhea, and osteoporosis [35]. Athletic amenorrhea results in an estrogen deficiency, which leads to increased bone resorption and decreased bone mass [24]. As a result, peak bone mass may not be achieved, and these women are at increased risk for future osteoporosis compared with someone who had achieved a higher peak bone mass by the third decade of life. Whereas boys generally enjoy the favorable effect of testosterone to build bone mass [24], adolescent girls with negative calcium balance and estrogen deficiency comprise a high-risk group for low peak bone mineral density and osteoporosis. Importantly, research has shown that dietary calcium intake at the recommended level protects from bone mineral density loss in women who take oral contraceptives [36].

In addition to future osteoporosis, calcium deficiency has been linked to an increased risk of fractures in adolescents, which may be something that they can more easily relate to than long-term risks [37]. Low calcium intake has also been associated with a possible increased risk of pre-eclampsia, colon cancer, and hypertension [24]. Adequate calcium not only maintains bone health in adolescence and beyond, but also seems to be protective against various diseases later in life. It is important to realize that calcium is not the only determinant of bone mass, especially in children and adolescents. Multiple studies have shown that regular physical activity is correlated with increased bone mineral content in boys and girls [38]. Weight-bearing exercise promotes growth in skeletal mass, especially before age 20, which can increase bone mass above genetically predetermined levels [39]. Although regular exercise is beneficial to bones, it is not known whether this can compensate for chronically low calcium intake, especially during puberty, when the growth rate is at its maximum.

Calcium supplementation is becoming increasingly common, especially in women, to augment dietary calcium intake and reach daily recommended levels. After a dietary analysis, if it is determined that adequate calcium cannot be obtained from food sources, supplementation is the next choice for meeting AI levels. The most common supplements—calcium carbonate and calcium citrate—are available in a variety of brand-name and generic forms and often include some amount of vitamin D. Calcium carbonate contains approximately 40% elemental calcium, whereas calcium citrate contains approximately 21%. The two have similar absorptive efficiencies in the gastrointestinal tract [26]. Doses should be kept to 500 mg or less, spread out over multiple times of day, to maximize each dose's absorption [40]. Supplementation has been shown to increase lumbar spine and total body bone mineral density in adolescent girls [41]. The effects of supplementation seem to be more beneficial in prepubertal than pubertal adolescents [42]. In adolescent athletes, this may lead to fewer stress fractures and less time lost to injury during training and competition.

Calcium is a vital nutrient for maintaining bone health and other bodily functions, such as muscle contraction, but most adolescents do not consume adequate amounts. Athletes, especially girls, are at risk for chronic calcium deficiency caused by caloric restriction to produce a leaner physique, which may be favorable in their sport. As such, it is essential to stress the importance of meeting the recommended daily calcium intake as an adolescent to prevent current and future problems that may be irreversible in adulthood.

Iron

Iron has multiple functions in the body, with approximately two thirds of the body's total iron present in hemoglobin to serve the oxygen delivery needs of body tissues. Approximately 4% of total iron is in myoglobin and 1% is in mitochondrial heme compounds, which promote intracellular oxidation and ATP production; 15% to 30% is stored as ferritin, primarily in the reticuloendothelial system and liver parenchymal cells [43].

Unlike other minerals, which have specific physiologic controls to regulate their concentration in the body, there is no mechanism for iron to alter its excretion; instead, total body iron is regulated at the level of intestinal absorption [43]. Healthy adults generally absorb 10% to 15% of dietary iron each day, but this can vary based on their individual iron status and the amount of plasma apotransferrin (a beta-globulin binding protein) available to bind dietary iron [44]. It is also important to recognize that not all dietary iron is equivalent. Heme iron is derived from hemoglobin, which is found largely in animal products, such as red meat, fish, and poultry. Nonheme iron is found in plant foods, such as lentils and beans, and is the form of iron used to fortify grain products [44]. Heme iron is much more efficiently absorbed from the gastrointestinal tract—at approximately 15% to 35%—and is independent of other foods in the diet. Nonheme iron is only approximately 2% to 20% absorbed, but this can be enhanced by concurrent consumption of meat protein and vitamin C. Conversely, nonheme iron absorption can be inhibited by calcium, tannins, polyphenols, phytates, and soy proteins, which presents a problem for vegetarians and individuals who restrict their meat intake to limit calories [45].

The RDA for iron, as determined by the US Food and Drug Administration, varies with gender and age. For boys, the RDA is 8 mg for ages 9 to 13 and 19 and older, but for ages 14 to 18 it increases to 11 mg/d. For girls, the RDA is 8 mg/d for ages 9 to 13, 15 mg/d for ages 14 to 18, and 18 mg/d for ages 19 to 50. Adolescents require a higher intake of iron to support growth, increases in lean body mass, and increases in blood volume [46]. They may have an inherent greater risk for iron deficiency compared with adults with similar iron consumption. For vegetarians who consume mostly nonheme iron along with substances that may inhibit its absorption, the RDA is nearly doubled to compensate for the reduced absorption efficiency in the gastrointestinal tract. For premenopausal vegetarian women, the RDA is 32 mg/d; for vegetarian men, the RDA rises to 14 mg/d. Iron consumption above 45 mg/d, the tolerable upper limit, can result in gastrointestinal distress [45].

Exercise can alter iron requirements and absorption, use, and loss. As such, iron deficiency and issues regarding iron supplementation in athletes are at the forefront of sports medicine research. Iron depletion occurs in three phases: depletion of iron stores, iron-deficient erythropoiesis, and iron-deficiency anemia. Complete depletion of iron stores is diagnosed by a serum ferritin level of less than 12 μg/L; values between 12 and 35 μg/L indicate partially exhausted iron stores. Iron-deficient erythropoiesis, also called iron deficiency without anemia, is characterized by increased concentrations of apotransferrin and decreased apotransferrin saturation with iron but normal hemoglobin levels. Anemia, the final state of iron deficiency, is diagnosed by microcytic hypochromic erythrocytes along with a hemoglobin level less than 12 g/dL in women and 13 g/dL in men [47]. One of the fundamental characteristics of anemia is that someone with even moderate iron-deficiency anemia may feel completely normal at rest; only during strenuous exercise are the effects of reduced oxygen-carrying capacity evident and the anemia "unmasked" [48].

Once it has been determined that an adolescent athlete has some form of iron depletion or deficiency, a nutritional analysis is helpful to locate ways to possibly get more iron from the diet. Five suggestions are (1) eating more lean red meat or dark poultry, (2) avoiding coffee or tea with meals, (3) drinking orange juice with breakfast, (4) cooking in cast-iron cookware, and (5) eating various foods in a "mixed" meal so as to enhance absorption of non-heme iron from grains and beans [49]. Depending on the severity of the iron deficiency, iron supplementation also may need to be started. The goal values are ferritin level more than 60 µg/L and hemoglobin level more than 12 g/dL. Nielsen and Nachtigall [50] recommend supplementing anyone with a ferritin level less than 35 µg/L, whereas Eichner [51] suggested algorithm for treatment of iron deficiency without anemia is as follows. For a ferritin level more than 40 µg/L, no treatment is necessary; for ferritin between 20 and 40 µg/L, take a daily multivitamin tablet that contains 27 mg elemental iron; for ferritin less than 20 µg/L, take one 325-mg tablet of ferrous sulfate (65 mg elemental iron) per day with dinner until all 100 tablets are gone. Ferritin levels then should be rechecked. For iron deficiency with anemia, two ferrous sulfate tablets per day are prescribed, with ferritin and hemoglobin levels rechecked after all 100 tablets are used. Usually a patient takes another course or two of 100 tablets to help build depleted iron stores [51]. On such a regimen, after an initial delay of a few days, hemoglobin should rise approximately 1 g/dL each week. It returns to a normal value within 2 months [49], although it may take up to 6 months to fully replenish iron stores [2]. As hemoglobin and ferritin are restored to acceptable values, the capacity for physical performance should concurrently increase back to pre-iron deficiency levels [48].

Many types of iron supplements are available, but they vary in the amount of elemental iron they contain. Deciding which iron supplement to use is heavily influenced by the degree of iron deficiency. Ferrous fumarate contains approximately 33% elemental iron, ferrous sulfate approximately 20% elemental iron, and ferrous gluconate approximately 12% [44]. Ferrous compounds are much more readily absorbed in the duodenum than ferric compounds [50]. Whereas iron supplements are widely used in women, they should not be given to men because of the risk for iron overload (leading to liver failure), which is more than twice the risk of iron deficiency in men [49]. Men and women are at risk for iron overload and hemochromatosis with iron supplementation. The incidence of homozygous hemochromatosis, an autosomal recessive disease in which patients absorb two to three times the normal amount of iron, is approximately 1:200 in the general population, whereas the heterozygous condition is much more common and may show no symptoms until iron supplementation is begun [52]. Genetic screening for the C282Y mutation in the hemochromatosis gene *HFE* is available and may be considered when a patient on iron supplementation presents with symptoms of iron overload, namely fatigue, weakness, weight loss, joint pain, and abdominal pain. If untreated, this condition may progress to liver fibrosis, cirrhosis, and eventually liver failure [52].

Iron deficiency in adolescent athletes, primarily girls, is an important condition that can have detrimental effects on performance and overall health if left untreated. Periodically screening female athletes and other endurance athletes may help to discover iron depletion before it reaches anemic levels, and dietary changes and supplementation can prevent significant decreases in exercise capacity for athletes.

Vitamin D

Vitamin D is an essential micronutrient that is involved in the regulation of plasma calcium levels and is necessary for overall bone health and a wide variety of other physiologic processes. Several sterol derivatives belong to the vitamin D family and perform essentially the same functions, albeit with different levels of potency depending on the specific nature of the compound. Vitamin D_3, also called cholecalciferol, can be obtained through the diet from animal products such as fish, eggs, and fortified milk, or through ultraviolet-B irradiation of 7-dehydrocholesterol, a compound normally found in the skin [23]. It is then transported to the liver, where it is hydroxylated to 25-$(OH)D_3$, or calcidiol [53], which is the most common circulating form of vitamin D and is generally used as a biochemical marker of vitamin D status [5]. Vitamin D_2, also called ergocalciferol, is obtained from plant foods in the diet or from ultraviolet irradiation of ergosterol. This form has several subtle chemical differences from D_3, which alter its metabolism and cause it to be somewhat less potent [54].

When the parathyroid gland senses low calcium in the extracellular fluid, PTH is released and causes conversion of 25-$(OH)D_3$ to 1,25-$(OH)_2D_3$ by 1α-hydroxylase (CYP27B1) within the proximal tubules of the kidney [53]. Absorption of calcium in the gastrointestinal tract depends on the availability of active 1,25-$(OH)_2D_3$, which increases production of a calcium-binding protein in intestinal epithelial cells; the rate of calcium absorption is directly proportional to the amount of this protein present [23]. Elevated 1,25-$(OH)_2D_3$ also causes increased resorption of bone since this active form is present in sufficient quantities, primarily when PTH is high, because plasma calcium is low and needs to be replenished. This increased calcium absorption and bone resorption form the basis for the "classical" biologic effects of vitamin D as a calciotropic hormone. 1,25-$(OH)_2D_3$ also promotes intestinal absorption of phosphate and decreases renal excretion of calcium and phosphate [23].

There is some debate over daily requirements and what constitutes "sufficient" serum 25-$(OH)D_3$ levels, especially in children and adolescents, in whom inadequate vitamin D may lead to lifelong skeletal abnormalities. The current AI guidelines for vitamin D are set at 200 IU (5 µg) for all individuals younger than age 50, but some question whether this is enough, especially for individuals who are not exposed to much sunlight [55]. It is fairly well known that a serum 25-(OH)D₃ level less than 12.5 nmol/L can lead to rickets in children and osteomalacia in adolescents and adults [56]. Levels less than 20 to 25 nmol/L may have detrimental effects on bone in the longer term, possibly leading to eventual bone disease [57], which is termed "subclinical vitamin D deficiency" [53]. Above this level, however, consequences become less well-defined; levels less than 50 nmol/L are generally classified as a "subclinical insufficiency" [53]. Both of these categories are in comparison to the severe clinical deficiency associated with rickets and osteomalacia. Subclinical vitamin D deficiency and insufficiency can be asymptomatic, or it may manifest as vague bone pain and tenderness [58]. Although the general lack of symptoms makes this deficiency seem harmless, it may lead to osteoporosis later in life [53]. In this borderline deficiency, the patient may still have normal or elevated plasma levels of 1,25-(OH)₂D₃ (likely caused by elevated PTH levels) despite already having the beginnings of osteomalacia [59]. Current literature estimates of adequate serum 25-(OH)D₃ levels for maintaining optimal bone health begin at 75 nmol/L, with the preferred amount being 90 to 100 nmol/L [60]. Some researchers also say that PTH levels should be measured along with 25-(OH)D₃ to keep PTH within the "normal" range, which is less than 53 pg/mL [58].

It is essential to realize that a large portion of the difficulty in setting sufficient vitamin D levels is caused by the fact that the "normal" value of vitamin D varies between populations based on geographic location and race and culture [58]. This is especially true for adolescent athletes. Athletes who live at more northern latitudes or who train primarily indoors, such as gymnasts, dancers, and figure skaters, are less likely to be getting sufficient vitamin D through UVB light conversion in the epidermis [2]. Darker races with more melanin in their skin have as much as a 50-fold decrease in the efficiency of dermal vitamin D conversion. Certain racial groups are inherently at greater risk for vitamin D deficiency than others [61]. Adolescent athletes who restrict their caloric intake to maintain a leaner physique are less likely to consume adequate vitamin D from the diet because of elimination of animal and dairy products. Compounding this deficiency is the fact that these same athletes are less likely to consume adequate calcium in their diet [2], the result of which may be failure to reach genetically programmed height and peak bone mineral density in the third decade of life [62]. Together, insufficient intake of vitamin D and calcium places these adolescents, particularly girls, at an increased risk for osteopenia and osteoporosis.

Vitamin D₃ also has a significant number of "nonclassical" actions in tissues besides bone that have received considerable attention in recent years. The receptor for 1,25-(OH)₂D₃, called VDR, is a transcription factor expressed in most tissues of the body; it complexes with another transcription factor, RXR, to activate vitamin D response elements in the promoter regions of target genes [54]. Loss of VDR causes alopecia, which implicates this molecule in normal hair follicle function. VDR can bind to β-catenin, a transcription factor in the Wnt pathway associated with several malignancies. It blocks the transcriptional activity of β-catenin and may partially explain the antiproliferative actions of 1,25-$(OH)_2D_3$ [54]. Vitamin D also plays a role in the regulation of cell growth, differentiation, and hormone secretion [62].

Although vitamin D has various beneficial effects in adults, especially in the prevention of chronic diseases (eg, hypertension, cancer, and cardiovascular disease), far less is known about the consequences of vitamin D deficiency in childhood and adolescence in relation to nonskeletal conditions. Research has shown that living at latitudes above 35° for the first decade of life doubles the risk for multiple sclerosis [63]. Vitamin D also plays an important immunosuppressive role in the body, although the exact mechanism is unclear [60]. Because of this, vitamin D deficiency has been implicated in various autoimmune diseases, including inflammatory bowel disease, rheumatoid arthritis, systemic lupus erythematosus, and type I diabetes mellitus [60]. A study of children in Finland who received 2000 IU (50 μg) of vitamin D daily during the first year of life showed an 80% reduction in the risk of developing type I diabetes [64].

It is difficult to determine the prevalence of subclinical vitamin D deficiency in the adolescent population because of the lack of solid cutoff values for serum 25-$(OH)D_3$ levels; however, a recent study estimated that only 50% of girls aged 9 to 13 years and 32% of girls aged 14 to 18 years meet the daily vitamin D recommendation of 200 IU [65]. The amount of 200 IU is only an AI amount, and it assumes some vitamin D attainment via dermal synthesis; evidence points to daily intakes higher than 200 IU as beneficial and possibly necessary during winter months or when sunlight exposure is minimal [53]. In the adolescent athlete population, the number who meet this daily requirement may be even lower because of indoor training or caloric restriction by elimination of animal and dairy products. Ways to improve vitamin D status include (1) increasing consumption of vitamin D-rich and fortified foods, (2) getting regular sunlight exposure, (3) supplementing with oral vitamin D and calcium, and (4) getting yearly vitamin D injections [58]. If diet and exposure to sun are insufficient to meet daily requirements, supplementation is the next alternative. Treatment for rickets and osteomalacia can involve up to 20,000 IU of vitamin D per day for several months, whereas subclinical vitamin D deficiency can be alleviated with much smaller doses. There is no set quantity for vitamin D supplementation caused by subclinical deficiency, but generally it should not exceed the tolerable upper limit of 2000 IU (50 μg) per day or toxicity and hypercalcemia may result [55].

Vitamin D is an essential—but often overlooked—micronutrient with various beneficial effects on bone health and the immune and cardiovascular systems. Although the AI level is set at 200 IU/d, many adolescents do not get this amount because of either dietary restrictions or lack of sun exposure. As such, it is often necessary to supplement vitamin D in the adolescent population to help prevent osteoporosis and a host of other chronic diseases later in life.

Fluid and electrolyte recommendations

Surprisingly, most athletes' fluid intake rarely balances sweat loss associated with exercise. Daily water balance depends on the net difference between water gain and water loss [66]. Total body water averages approximately 60% of body mass, with a range of approximately 45% to 75% [66]. These differences are primarily caused by body composition; fat-free mass is approximately 70% to 80% water, whereas adipose tissue is approximately 10% water [66]. Athletes can monitor their hydration status by using simple urine and body weight measurements. A morning nude body weight is usually stable and fluctuates less than 1% [67–70]. A baseline value typically can be made after three consecutive measurements [71]. Urine specific gravity of 1.020 or less indicates euhydration [72–74]. Urine osmolarity values of 700 mOsmol/kg^{-1} or less indicate euhydration [72,74,75].

Dehydration increases physiologic strain and perceived effort to perform the same exercise task, which is accentuated in warm and hot weather [76]. Dehydration ($>2\%$ body weight) can degrade aerobic exercise performance and cognitive/mental performance, especially in warm or hot weather [66,77,78]. The greater the dehydration level, the greater the physiologic strain and aerobic exercise performance decrement [66]. Dehydration (3% body weight) has marginal influence on degrading aerobic exercise performance when cold stress is present [66,79–81]. Dehydration (3%–5% body weight) does not degrade either anaerobic performance or muscular strength [66,82,83]. Hyperhydration does not provide any thermoregulatory advantages [84] but can delay the onset of dehydration [85].

The goal of drinking during exercise is to prevent excessive ($>2\%$ body weight loss from water deficit) dehydration and excessive changes in electrolyte balance to avert compromised performance. The American College of Sports Medicine and National Association of Athletic Trainers recommend drinking 14 to 20 oz (400–600 mL) of fluid 2 to 3 hours before exercise [86,87]. The concept behind this practice is that hydration will be optimal yet allow enough time for excess fluid to be excreted as urine before competition or exercise begins. Athletes also should be well hydrated and drink generous amounts of fluid 24 hours before exercising [2].

For optimal performance, it is recommended that athletes consume at least 6 to 12 oz (150–350 mL) of fluid at 15- to 20-minute intervals, beginning at the start of exercise [86,87]. For events that last longer that 1 hour, fluids that contain carbohydrates in concentrations of 4% to 8% are recommended, although these types of fluid can be used for events that last less than 1 hour [86].

Athletes should not rely on thirst as an indicator that they need to drink after exercise. Fluid intake after exercise is necessary to replace losses incurred during the activity, which rarely occurs voluntarily. Body weight changes are the best method of determining fluid replacement amounts after exercise. In general, 500 mL of fluid should be consumed for every 1 lb of weight lost; for each kilogram lost, approximately 1.5 L of fluid should be consumed [88]. In the 2 to 4 hours after exercise, athletes should make a conscience effort to replace fluid losses with a volume equivalent to 150% of the weight loss [89]. Including sodium either in or with fluids consumed after exercise reduces the diuresis that occurs when only plain water is ingested [87,90]. Sodium also helps the rehydration process by maintaining plasma osmolality and the desire to drink. Because most commercial sport drinks do not contain enough sodium to optimize postexercise fluid replacement, athletes can rehydrate in conjunction with a sodium-containing meal [91]. High sodium items include soups, pickles, cheeses, processed meats, pizza, pretzels, and popcorn. Using condiments such as soy sauce and ketchup and salting food at the table also increase sodium intake [2].

Adequate fluid intake and prevention of dehydration are especially important for children and adolescents. For several reasons, they are more at risk for developing dehydration and hyperthermia. They have fewer sweat glands and sweat less per gland, which decreases their capacity to dissipate heat through evaporation. They experience greater heat production during exercise but have less ability to transfer heat from the muscle to skin. They also have a greater body surface area that can result in excessive heat gain in extreme heat and excessive heat loss in the cold. They also have a lower cardiac output, which reduces their capacity for heat transport from the core to the skin during strenuous exercise. Finally, they acclimatize to exercising in the heat more gradually than adults. A young adolescent may require five to six sessions to achieve the same degree of acclimatization acquired by an adult in two to three sessions in the same environment [92,93].

Certain medical conditions that affect children and adolescents put them at higher risk for developing heat-related illnesses. Excessive fluid loss may occur with fever, gastroenteritis, congenital heart disease, obesity, or bulimia. Obesity is associated with an increased risk of heat-related illness compared with normal weight children and adolescents for several reasons. Only a small amount of heat is needed to increase the temperature of a large amount of fat mass. Fat mass has lower water content than lean body mass (so a greater amount of fluid is lost in persons with high fat mass). Obese children expend greater effort than lean children, given the same intensity of exercise, which increases their overall body temperature more quickly [93].

Ergogenic aids

Ergogenic aids *claim* to increase strength, performance, and lean muscle mass. It is estimated that sales of nutritional supplements are as high as

$12 million in the United States [94]. The portion of these sales that are for adolescents and children is unknown but is estimated to be significant because purchase is available over the counter in most cases. In the United States, the Dietary Supplement Health and Education Act of 1994 [95] allows supplement manufacturers to make claims regarding the effect of products on the structure/function of the body, as long as they do not claim to "diagnose, mitigate, treat, cure or prevent" a specific disease. As long as a special supplement label indicates the active ingredients and the entire ingredient list is provided, claims of enhanced performance—valid or not—can be made. The US Food and Drug Administration does not regulate these products.

Creatine

Creatine is one of the most popular nutritional supplements, with yearly sales over $300 million in the United States according to the *Nutritional Business Journal*. No studies have shown this supplement to be safe in people younger than 18 years or have shown that it has an ergogenic effect [96]. Its use is increasing in the younger population, however [96]. Finally, the American College of Sports Medicine does not recommend and discourages creatine use in people younger than 18 years old because of unknown potential adverse health effects [97]. Creatine is not banned by the National Collegiate Athletic Association (NCAA), International Olympic Committee (IOC), or major league sports.

Creatine is naturally formed by the combination of glycine, arginine, and methionine [98]. Creatine is produced in physiologic (1 g/d) amounts by the kidney, liver, and pancreas and stored in skeletal muscle. These stores are broken down at a relatively constant rate of 2 g/dL into creatinine, which is excreted in the kidney. The daily recommendation for creatine is 2 g/d; 1 g/d must come from dietary sources. Dietary sources of creatine include meat and fish [98].

Common side effects associated with creatine use in adults include weight gain, muscle cramps, diarrhea, abdominal pain, and nausea. Creatine is also perceived to cause dehydration; however, no study to date has demonstrated this in athletes. There are two cases of adult-onset renal failure in creatine users, although there were several confounding variables in these situations [99,100].

In a recent middle and high school study, Metzel [101] examined the frequency and demographics of creatine use in 1103 participants in a suburb of New York City. He found that creatine is being used by middle and high school athletes at all grade levels [101]. The highest prevalence was in grade 12 (44%) and the lowest in grade 7 (2.1%) [101]. Use was significantly more common among boys (8.8%) than girls (1.8%). Creatine use also was found to be more common among football players, wrestlers, hockey players, gymnasts, and lacrosse players. The most common reasons cited for taking creatine were enhanced performance (74%) and improved appearance (61%) [101].

Androstenedione

Androstenedione is a steroid prohormone, a precursor to testosterone that is thought to work by being degraded into free testosterone. Most well-designed studies show no increase in testosterone concentrations with supplementation with androstenedione [102–106]. What is interesting is that several of the studies have shown an increase in estrogen, which is associated with an increase in fat mass, not lean muscle mass. No studies have shown an increase in performance or lean body mass [103,106]. Side effects of androstenedione include a reduction in high-density lipoprotein and down-regulation of endogenous testosterone synthesis [103,104,107]. A Canadian study showed that 1.7% of adolescent boys and 0% of adolescent girls used androstenedione [108]. Currently, androstenedione is banned by the IOC, NCAA, National Football League, and Major League Baseball and is available as an over-the-counter nutritional supplement.

Growth hormone

Human growth hormone (GH) is an endogenous peptide secreted by the anterior pituitary gland. It functions primarily in an anabolic way, increasing amino acid uptake and protein synthesis and supporting other growth-promoting functions. Much of the basic science of GH remains unknown. Secretion of GH is regulated by several factors, including GH-releasing hormone, sleep, exercise, L-dopa, and arginine [109,110]. No studies have revealed that GH increases performance; however, it does have a repartitions effect, which decreases subcutaneous fat, making individuals appear more toned [111–114]. High levels of GH can lead to myopathic muscle changes, water retention, and carpal tunnel syndrome [110,115]. Additional risks include premature physeal closure, jaw enlargement, hypertension, and slipped femoral capital epiphysis [116,117]. Severe but rare side effects include papilledema with intracranial hypertension [118].

In an American high school study by Rickert [119], 5% of the boys reported using GH, with ten students indicating explicitly that it was for improving sports performance. The latest NCAA study found that 3.5% of athletes reported using GH in the past 12 months [120]. GH is banned by all major sporting leagues; however, no reliable test to detect use by athletes has been developed.

Ephedrine-type alkaloids

Ephedrine is a stimulant with a chemical structure similar to catecholamines. It is derived from the herb known as ma huang or guarana. It stimulates the release of norepinephrine, which results in vasoconstriction and increased blood pressure similar to amphetamines. Limited studies have shown that ephedrine may increase performance [121,122]. A study by Chandler revealed that dexedrine improved quadriceps strength and anaerobic capacity. It also showed an increase time to exhaustion [121]. Gill showed that pseudoephedrine increased peak power during cycling and improved lung function [122]. Side effects from amphetamines are serious and include hypertension, ventricular arrhythmias, hallucination, seizures, paranoid psychoses, myocardial infarction, and death [100,123].

In an American high school study that included 270 athletes, Kayton [124] showed that 26% of girls and 12% of boys had tried ephedrine-type products. The NCAA reported that 3.9% of the athletes had tried ephedrine in 2001. The most recent study by the NCAA in 2004 showed that 38% of Division I ice hockey teams surveyed used ephedrine and 46% used pseudoephedrine with the intention of increasing performance [125]. The US Food and Drug Administration removed ephedrine from the market in 2004. Ephedrine products are banned by the IOC, NCAA, Major League Baseball, National Basketball Association, and the National Football League.

Summary

Proper nutrition and hydration are important for all athletes. Children and adolescents have unique nutritional requirements depending on age, level of maturity, growth rate, and energy expenditure. Supplement use is increasing in all groups despite significant known side effects and little data to support an increase in performance.

References

[1] The energy yielding nutrients: carbohydrates, protein and fat. In: Ruud JS, editor. Nutrition and the female athlete. New York: CRC Press, Inc.; 1996. p. 22–50.

[2] American College of Sports Medicine, American Dietetic Association, and Dietitians of Canada. Joint position statement: nutrition and athletic performance. Med Sci Sports Exerc 2000;32(12):2130–45.

[3] Bonci L. Nutrition. In: McKeag DB. Moeller JL, editors. ACSM primary care in sports medicine. 2nd edition. Philadelphia: Lippincott Williams and Wilkins; 2007. p. 35–52.

[4] Powers SK, Howley ET, editors. Exercise physiology: theory and application to fitness and performance. 5th edition. New York: McGraw-Hill Co.; 2004. p. 458–78.

[5] Dietary reference intake for calcium, phosphorus, magnesium, vitamin D and fluoride. In: Institute of Medicine, editor. Nutrition and the female athlete. Washington, DC: National Academies Press; 1989. p. 71–145.

[6] Dietary references intake for thiamin, riboflavin, niacin, vitamin B6, folate, vitamin B12, pentothenic acid, biotin and chlorine. In: Institute of Medicine, editor. Nutrition and the female athlete. Washington, DC: National Academies Press; 1989.

[7] Juzwiak CR, Paschoal VC, Lopez FA. [Nutrition and physical activity]. J Pediatr (Rio J) 2000;76(Suppl 3):S349–58.

[8] Dietary carbohydrates: sugars and starches. In: Institute of Medicine, editor. Dietary reference intakes for energy, carbohydrates, fiber, fat, fatty acids, cholesterol, protein and amino acids. Washington, DC: National Academies Press; 2002. p. 265–338.

[9] Spear B. Sports nutrition. In: Stang J, Story M, editors. Guidelines for adolescent nutrition services. Minneapolis, MN. p. 199–208.

[10] Berning JR. Nutrition for exercise and sports performance. In: Mahan LK, Escott-Stump S, editors. Krause's food, nutrition & diet therapy. Philadelphia: W.B. Saunders Co.; 2000. p. 534–57.

[11] Earnest C. Preventing nutritional disorders in athletes: focus on the basics. Curr Sports Med Rep 2002;1(3):172–8.

[12] Ahlborg B, Bergstrom J, Ekelund LC, et al. Muscle glycogen and muscle electrolytes during prolonged physical exercise. Acta Physiol Scand 1967;70:129–42.

[13] Cataletto M, Birrer R, Griesemer B. Nutrition: sports medicine board review (pearls of wisdom). New York: McGraw-Hill Co.; 2006. p. 81–9.

[14] Apex Fitness Group. Nutritional concerns for the young athlete: part II. Available at: www. ptonthenet.com. Accessed June 14, 2007.

[15] DiMarco NM, Essery EV. Nutrition. In: O'Connor F, Sallis R, Wilder R, et al, editors. Sports medicine: just the facts. New York: McGraw-Hill; 2004. p. 83–90.

[16] Tarnopolsky LJ, MacDougall JD, Atkinson SA, et al. Gender differences in substrate for endurance exercise. J Appl Physiol 1990;68(1):302–8.

[17] VanHeest J, Mahoney C. Female athletes: factors impacting successful performance. Curr Sports Med Rep 2007;6(3):190–4.

[18] Ruby BC, Roberg RA. Gender differences in substrate utilisation during exercise. Sports Med 1994;17(6):393–410.

[19] Petrie HJ, Stover EA, Horswill CA. Nutritional concerns for the child and adolescent competitor. Nutrition 2004;20(7–8):620–31.

[20] Volpe SL. A nutritionist's view: young athletes' nutritional needs for optimal performance. American College of Sports Medicine's Health & Fitness Journal 2006;10(5):30–1.

[21] Unnithan VB, Goulopoulou S. Nutrition for the pediatric athlete. Curr Sports Med Rep 2004;3(4):206–11.

[22] Sherman WM, Brodowicz G, Wright DA, et al. Effects of 4 h preexercise carbohydrate feedings on cycling performance. Med Sci Sports Exerc 1989;21(5):598–604.

[23] Thomas DE, Brotherhood JR, Brand JC. Carbohydrate feeding before exercise: effect of glycemic index. Int J Sports Med 1991;12(2):180–6.

[24] Burke LM, Collier GR, Hargreaves M. Muscle glycogen storage after prolonged exercise: effect of the glycemic index of carbohydrate feedings. J Appl Physiol 1993;75(2): 1019–23.

[25] Guyton AC, Hall JE. Parathyroid hormone, calcitonin, calcium and phosphate metabolism, vitamin D, bone and teeth. Textbook of Medical Physiology. Philadelphia: Saunders; 2005. p. 978–92.

[26] NIH Consensus conference. Optimal calcium intake: NIH consensus development panel on optimal calcium intake. JAMA 1994;272(24):1942–8.

[27] Office of Dietary Supplements. NIH Clinical Center National Institutes of Health. Dietary supplement fact sheet: calcium. Available at: http://dietary-supplements.info.nih.gov/ factsheets/calcium.asp. Accessed June 25, 2007.

[28] Tanner J, editor. Growth at adolescence. 2nd edition. Oxford (UK): Blackwell Publishers Ltd; 1962. p. 1–8.

[29] Abrams SA, Stuff JE. Calcium metabolism in girls: current dietary intakes lead to low rates of calcium absorption and retention during puberty. Am J Clin Nutr 1994;60(5):739–43.

[30] Steingrimsdottir L, Gunnarsson O, Indridason OS, et al. Relationship between serum parathyroid hormone levels, vitamin D sufficiency, and calcium intake. JAMA 2005;294(18): 2336–41.

[31] Subar AF, Krebs-Smith SM, Cook A, et al. Dietary sources of nutrients among US adults, 1989 to 1991. J Am Diet Assoc 1998;98(5):537–47.

[32] Zemel MB, Thompson W, Milstead A, et al. Calcium and dairy acceleration of weight and fat loss during energy restriction in obese adults. Obes Res 2004;12(4):582–90.

[33] NIH News Release. "Calcium crisis" affects American youth: expanded Web site seeks to inform children of dangers of low calcium intake. Available at: http://www.nih.gov/news/pr/dec2001/nichd-10.htm. Accessed June 25, 2007.

[34] Hansen MA, Overgaard K, Riis BJ, et al. Role of peak bone mass and bone loss in postmenopausal osteoporosis: 12 year study. BMJ 1991;303(6808):961–4.

[35] Otis CL, Drinkwater B, Johnson M, et al. American College of Sports Medicine position stand: the female athlete triad. Med Sci Sports Exerc 1997;29(5):1669–71.

[36] Teegarden D, Legowski P, Gunther CW, et al. Dietary calcium intake protects women consuming oral contraceptives from spine and hip bone loss. J Clin Endocrinol Metab 2005; 90(9):5127–33.

[37] Baker SS, Cochran WJ, Flores CA, et al. American Academy of Pediatrics Committee on Nutrition: calcium requirements of infants, children, and adolescents. Pediatrics 1999; 104(5 Pt 1):1152–7.

[38] Bradney M, Pearce G, Naughton G, et al. Moderate exercise during growth in prepubertal boys: changes in bone mass, size, volumetric density, and bone strength: a controlled prospective study. J Bone Miner Res 1998;13(12):1814–21.

[39] Turner CH. Site-specific skeletal effects of exercise: importance of interstitial fluid pressure. Bone 1999;24(3):161–2.

[40] National Institute of Arthritis and Musculoskeletal and Skin Diseases. Calcium supplements: what to look for. Available at: http://www.niams.nih.gov/bone/hi/calcium_supp.htm. Accessed June 25, 2007.

[41] Lloyd T, Andon MB, Rollings N, et al. Calcium supplementation and bone mineral density in adolescent girls. JAMA 1993;270(7):841–4.

[42] Javaid MK, Cooper C. Prenatal and childhood influences on osteoporosis. Best Pract Res Clin Endocrinol Metab 2002;16(2):349–67.

[43] Guyton AC, Hall JE. Red blood cells, anemia, and polycythemia. Textbook of medical physiology. Philadelphia: Saunders; 2005. p. 424–8.

[44] Office of Dietary Supplements. NIH Clinical Center National Institutes of Health. Dietary supplementation fact sheet: iron. Available at: http://dietary-supplements.info.nih.gov/factsheets/iron.asp#en33. Accessed June 18, 2007.

[45] Institute of Medicine. Dietary reference intakes: for vitamin A, vitamin K, arsenic, boron, chromium, copper, iodine, iron, manganese, molybdenum, nickel, silicon, vanadium, and zinc. Washington, DC: National Academies Press; 2002. p. 290–393.

[46] Sinclair LM, Hinton PS. Prevalence of iron deficiency with and without anemia in recreationally active men and women. J Am Diet Assoc 2005;105(6):975–8.

[47] Akabas SR, Dolins KR. Micronutrient requirements of physically active women: what can we learn from iron? Am J Clin Nutr 2005;81(5):1246S–51S.

[48] Eichner ER, Scott WA. Exercise as disease detector. Phys Sportsmed 1998;26(3):41–52.

[49] Eichner ER. Anemia and blood boosting. Sports Science Exchange 2001;14(2):81–4.

[50] Nielsen P, Nachtigall D. Iron supplementation in athletes: current recommendations. Sports Medicine 1998;26(4):207–16.

[51] Eichner ER. Coping with anemia. Sports Medicine Digest 2000;22(5):57–8.

[52] Ajioka RS, Kushner JP. Clinical consequences of iron overload in hemochromatosis homozygotes. Blood 2003;101(9):3351–3.

[53] Cashman KD. Vitamin D in childhood and adolescence. Postgrad Med J 2007;83(978): 230–5.

[54] Bikle DD. What is new in vitamin D: 2006–2007. Curr Opin Rheumatol 2007;19(4): 383–8.

[55] National Institutes of Health. Medline plus drugs and supplements: vitamin D. Available at: http://www.nlm.nih.gov/medlineplus/druginfo/natural/patient-vitamind.html. Accessed July 3, 2007.

[56] Pedersen P, Michaelsen KF, Molgaard C. Children with nutritional rickets referred to hospitals in Copenhagen during a 10-year period. Acta Paediatr 2003;92(1):87–90.

[57] Basha B, Rao DS, Han ZH, et al. Osteomalacia due to vitamin D depletion: a neglected consequence of intestinal malabsorption. Am J Med 2000;108(4):296–300.

[58] Masud F. Vitamin D levels for optimum bone health. Singapore Med J 2007;48(3):207–12.

[59] Lips P. Vitamin D deficiency and secondary hyperparathyroidism in the elderly: consequences for bone loss and fractures and therapeutic implications. Endocr Rev 2001; 22(4):477–501.

[60] Arnson Y, Amital H, Shoenfeld Y. Vitamin D and autoimmunity: new etiological and therapeutical considerations. Ann Rheum Dis 2007;0:1–6.

[61] Holick MF. The UV advantage: the medical breakthrough that shows how to harness the power of the sun for your health. New York: ibooks; 2003.

[62] Holick MF. Sunlight and vitamin D for bone health and prevention of autoimmune diseases, cancers, and cardiovascular disease. Am J Clin Nutr 2004;80(Suppl 6):1678S–88S.

[63] Holick MF. Resurrection of vitamin D deficiency and rickets. J Clin Invest 2006;116(8): 2062–72.

[64] Hypponen E, Laara E, Reunanen A, et al. Intake of vitamin D and risk of type 1 diabetes: a birth-cohort study. Lancet 2001;358(9292):1500–3.

[65] Moore C, Murphy MM, Keast DR, et al. Vitamin D intake in the United States. J Am Diet Assoc 2004;104(6):980–3.

[66] Institute of Medicine. Water: dietary reference intakes for water, sodium, chloride, potassium and sulfate. Washington, DC: National Academies Press; 2005. p. 73–185.

[67] Adolph E, editor. Physiological regulations. Lancaster (PA): The Jacques Cattell Press; 1943. p. 88–92.

[68] Cheuvront SN, Carter R III, Montain SJ, et al. Daily body mass variability and stability in active men undergoing exercise-heat stress. Int J Sport Nutr Exerc Metab 2004;14(5): 532–40.

[69] Grandjean AC, Reimers KJ, Bannick KE, et al. The effect of caffeinated, non-caffeinated, caloric and non-caloric beverages on hydration. J Am Coll Nutr 2000;19(5):591–600.

[70] Grandjean AC, Reimers KJ, Haven MC, et al. The effect on hydration of two diets, one with and one without plain water. J Am Coll Nutr 2003;22(2):165–73.

[71] Sawka MN, Burke LM, Eichner ER, et al. American College of Sports Medicine position stand: exercise and fluid replacement. Med Sci Sports Exerc 2007;39(2):377–90.

[72] Armstrong S, Maresh CM, Castellani JW, et al. Urinary indices of hydration status. Int J Sport Nutr 1994;4:265–79.

[73] Bartok C, Schoeller DA, Sullivan JC, et al. Hydration testing in collegiate wrestlers undergoing hypertonic dehydration. Med Sci Sports Exerc 2004;36(3):510–7.

[74] Popowski LA, Oppliger RA, Patrick LG, et al. Blood and urinary measures of hydration status during progressive acute dehydration. Med Sci Sports Exerc 2001;33(5):747–53.

[75] Shirreffs SM, Maughan RJ. Urine osmolality and conductivity as indices of hydration status in athletes in the heat. Med Sci Sports Exerc 1998;30(11):1598–602.

[76] Sawka MN, Coyle EF. Influence of body water and blood volume on thermoregulation and exercise performance in the heat. Exerc Sport Sci Rev 1999;27:167–218.

[77] Casa DJ, Clarkson PM, Roberts WO. American College of Sports Medicine roundtable on hydration and physical activity: consensus statements. Curr Sports Med Rep 2005;4(3): 115–27.

[78] Cheuvront SN, Carter R III, Sawka MN. Fluid balance and endurance exercise performance. Curr Sports Med Rep 2003;2(4):202–8.

[79] Cheuvront SN, Carter R III, Castellani JW, et al. Hypohydration impairs endurance exercise performance in temperate but not cold air. J Appl Physiol 2005;99(5):1972–6.

[80] Cheuvront SN, Carter R III, Haymes EM, et al. No effect of moderate hypohydration or hyperthermia on anaerobic exercise performance. Med Sci Sports Exerc 2006;38(6): 1093–7.

[81] Jacobs I. The effects of thermal dehydration on performance of the Wingate anaerobic test. Int J Sport Nutr 1980;1:21–4.

[82] Evetovich TK, Boyd JC, Drake SM, et al. Effect of moderate dehydration on torque, electromyography, and mechanomyography. Muscle Nerve 2002;26(2):225–31.

[83] Greiwe JS, Staffey KS, Melrose DR, et al. Effects of dehydration on isometric muscular strength and endurance. Med Sci Sports Exerc 1998;30(2):284–8.

[84] Latzka WA, Sawka MN, Montain SJ, et al. Hyperhydration: thermoregulatory effects during compensable exercise-heat stress. J Appl Physiol 1997;83(3):860–6.

[85] Latzka WA, Sawka MN, Montain SJ, et al. Hyperhydration: tolerance and cardiovascular effects during uncompensable exercise-heat stress. J Appl Physiol 1998;84(6): 1858–64.

[86] Convertino VA, Armstrong LE, Coyle EF, et al. American College of Sports Medicine position stand: exercise and fluid replacement. Med Sci Sports Exerc 1996;28(1):i–vii.

[87] Casa DJ, Armstrong LE, Hillman SK, et al. National athletic trainers' association position statement: fluid replacement for athletes. J Athl Train 2000;35(2):212–24.

[88] Roy BD, Tarnopolsky MA, MacDougall JD, et al. Effect of glucose supplement timing on protein metabolism after resistance training. J Appl Physiol 1997;82(6):1882–8.

[89] Shirreffs SM, Taylor AJ, Leiper JB, et al. Post-exercise rehydration in man: effects of volume consumed and drink sodium content. Med Sci Sports Exerc 1996;28(10): 1260–71.

[90] Maughan RJ, Leiper JB. Sodium intake and post-exercise rehydration in man. Eur J Appl Physiol Occup Physiol 1995;71(4):311–9.

[91] Maughan RJ, Leiper JB, Shirreffs SM. Restoration of fluid balance after exercise-induced dehydration: effects of food and fluid intake. Eur J Appl Physiol Occup Physiol 1996; 73(3–4):317–25.

[92] Steen SN. Timely statement of The American Dietetic Association: nutrition guidance for adolescent athletes in organized sports. J Am Diet Assoc 1996;96(6):611–2.

[93] Spear B. Nutrition in adolescence. In: Mahan LK, Escott-Stump S, editors. Krause's food, nutrition and diet therapy. Philadelphia: W.B. Saunders Company; 2000. p. 257–70.

[94] Leder BZ, Catlin DH, Longcope C, et al. Metabolism of orally administered androstenedione in young men. J Clin Endocrinol Metab 2001;86(8):3654–8.

[95] 103rd Congress. Public law 103–417. Dietary supplements health and Education Act of 1994. (21USC 3419(r)(6)).

[96] Metzl JD. Strength training and nutritional supplement use in adolescents. Curr Opin Pediatr 1999;11(4):292–6.

[97] Terjung RL, Clarkson P, Eichner ER, et al. American College of Sports Medicine round-table: the physiological and health effects of oral creatine supplementation. Med Sci Sports Exerc 2000;32(3):706–17.

[98] Balsom PD, Soderlund K, Ekblom B. Creatine in humans with special reference to creatine supplementation. Sports Med 1994;18(4):268–80.

[99] Pritchard NR, Kalra PA. Renal dysfunction accompanying oral creatine supplements. Lancet 1998;351(9111):1252–3.

[100] Koshy KM, Griswold E, Schneeberger EE. Interstitial nephritis in a patient taking creatine. N Engl J Med 1999;340(10):814–5.

[101] Metzl JD, Small E, Levine SR, et al. Creatine use among young athletes. Pediatrics 2001; 108(2):421–5.

[102] Ballantyne CS, Phillips SM, MacDonald JR, et al. The acute effects of androstenedione supplementation in healthy young males. Can J Appl Physiol 2000;25(1):68–78.

[103] Broeder CE, Quindry J, Brittingham K, et al. The Andro project: physiological and hormonal influences of androstenedione supplementation in men 35 to 65 years old participating in a high-intensity resistance training program. Arch Intern Med 2000;160(20): 3093–104.

[104] King DS, Sharp RL, Vukovich MD, et al. Effect of oral androstenedione on serum testosterone and adaptations to resistance training in young men: a randomized controlled trial. JAMA 1999;281(21):2020–8.

[105] Rasmussen BB, Volpi E, Gore DC, et al. Androstenedione does not stimulate muscle protein anabolism in young healthy men. J Clin Endocrinol Metab 2000;85(1):55–9.

[106] Wallace MB, Lim J, Cutler A, et al. Effects of dehydroepiandrosterone vs androstenedione supplementation in men. Med Sci Sports Exerc 1999;31(12):1788–92.

[107] Brown GA, Vukovich MD, Martini ER, et al. Endocrine and lipid responses to chronic androstenediol-herbal supplementation in 30 to 58 year old men. J Am Coll Nutr 2001; 20(5):520–8.

[108] Bell A, Dorsch KD, McCreary DR, et al. A look at nutritional supplement use in adolescents. J Adolesc Health 2004;34(6):508–16.

[109] Williams MH, Branch JD. Ergogenic aids for improved performance. In: Garrett WE, Kirkendall DT, editors. Exercise and sport science. Philadelphia: Lippincott, Williams and Wilkins; 2000. p. 373–84.

[110] Tokish JM, Kocher MS, Hawkins RJ. Ergogenic aids: a review of basic science, performance, side effects, and status in sports. Am J Sports Med 2004;32(6):1543–53.

[111] Frisch H. Growth hormone and body composition in athletes. J Endocrinol Invest 1999; 22(Suppl 5):106–9.

[112] Taaffe DR, Pruitt L, Reim J, et al. Effect of recombinant human growth hormone on the muscle strength response to resistance exercise in elderly men. J Clin Endocrinol Metab 1994;79(5):1361–6.

[113] Yarasheski KE. Growth hormone effects on metabolism, body composition, muscle mass, and strength. Exerc Sport Sci Rev 1994;22:285–312.

[114] Rennie MJ. Claims for the anabolic effects of growth hormone: a case of the emperor's new clothes? Br J Sports Med 2003;37(2):100–5.

[115] MacIntyre JG. Growth hormone and athletes. Sports Med 1987;4(2):129–42.

[116] Williams MH, editor. The ergogenic edge: pushing the limits of sports performance. Champaign (IL): Human Kinetics Publishers; 1997. p. 213–5.

[117] Calfee R, Fadale P. Popular ergogenic drugs and supplements in young athletes. Pediatrics 2006;117(3):e577–89.

[118] McDevitt ER. Ergogenic drugs in sports. In: DeLee J, Drez D, editors. Orthopaedic sports medicine: principles and practice. Philadelphia: WB Saunders; 2002. p. 471–83.

[119] Rickert VI, Pawlak-Morello C, Sheppard V, et al. Human growth hormone: a new substance of abuse among adolescents? Clin Pediatr (Phila) 1992;31(12):723–6.

[120] NCAA study of substance use habits of college student-athletes; 2001. Available at: www. ncaa.org/library/research.html#substance_use_habits. Accessed January 20, 2006.

[121] Chandler JV, Blair SN. The effect of amphetamines on selected physiological components related to athletic success. Med Sci Sports Exerc 1980;12(1):65–9.

[122] Gill ND, Shield A, Blazevich AJ, et al. Muscular and cardiorespiratory effects of pseudoephedrine in human athletes. Br J Clin Pharmacol 2000;50(3):205–13.

[123] Haller CA, Benowitz NL. Adverse cardiovascular and central nervous system events associated with dietary supplements containing ephedra alkaloids. N Engl J Med 2000; 343(25):1833–8.

[124] Nissen S, Sharp RL, Panton L, et al. Beta-hydroxy-beta-methylbutyrate (HMB) supplementation in humans is safe and may decrease cardiovascular risk factors. J Nutr 2000; 130(8):1937–45.

[125] Videman T, Lereim I, Hemmingsson P, et al. Changes in hemoglobin values in elite cross-country skiers from 1987–1999. Scand J Med Sci Sports 2000;10(2):98–102.

ELSEVIER
SAUNDERS

Phys Med Rehabil Clin N Am
19 (2008) 399–418

PHYSICAL MEDICINE
AND REHABILITATION
CLINICS OF
NORTH AMERICA

Psychologic Stress Related to Injury and Impact on Sport Performance

Angela H. Nippert, PhD[a,*],
Aynsley M. Smith, RN, PhD[b,c]

[a]*Department of Kinesiology and Health Sciences, Concordia University-St. Paul,
275 Syndicate Street North, St. Paul, MN 55104, USA*
[b]*Mayo Clinic Sports Medicine Center, Mayo Clinic, 200 First Street Southwest,
Rochester, MN 55905, USA*
[c]*Department of Orthopedic Surgery and Physical Medicine and Rehabilitation,
Mayo Medical School, 200 First Street Southwest, Rochester, MN 55905, USA*

Injury rates are high among children and adolescent athletes. Psychosocial stressors, such as personality, history of stressors, and life event stress can influence injury occurrence. After injury, athletic identity, self-esteem, and significant others—such as parents, coaches, and teammates—can affect injury recovery and sport performance. Goal setting, positive self-talk, attribution theory, and relaxation or mental imagery are psychologic interventions that can help injured athletes cope with psychosocial stressors. Medical professionals should be aware of the potential influence that psychosocial stressors and psychologic interventions can have on injury occurrence, injury recovery, and sport performance.

M.B, a 14 year old white, athletic basketball player suffered severe ankle sprains while attending a parochial school. Before these injuries, M.B. was dealing with his parents' impending divorce. Although the divorce was stressful, he felt he had a strong support system from his teammates. Moreover, M.B., a high athletic identity player with high self-esteem, had been identified as a promising, talented point guard. Perhaps related to the ankle sprains, the following season he was troubled by severe Achilles tendonitis and was unable to participate a full season. Feeling depressed, frustrated, misunderstood by the coach, alienated from his team, and without any known coping skills other than sport affiliation, M.B. began to hang out with a different peer group. Bored and feeling worthless, he

* Corresponding author.
E-mail address: nippert@csp.edu (A.H. Nippert).

1047-9651/08/$ - see front matter © 2008 Elsevier Inc. All rights reserved.
doi:10.1016/j.pmr.2007.12.003

doubted his physicians and physical therapists in terms of their ability to help him get back into sports and into the line up. As a result, he started to sever his connection to basketball.

M.B. replaced his athleticism with risk taking in the party scene: substituting the "high" of athletic competition and success with experimental highs from pot, alcohol, and sex.

M.B. continued to see his sport psychology counselor, who expressed concern about him giving up on his rehabilitation. He went snowboarding a few times, which did not seem to aggravate his Achilles tendonitis symptoms. In doing so, he gradually felt reconnected with his athleticism. Together, M.B. and the counselor wrote a script for a DVD to be used to warn other adolescents about the psychosocial pitfalls of unresolved sport injury. M.B. embraced this challenge and gradually became a role model, "walking the talk" for more optimal behavior. His self-esteem increased by doing something that would help others. Gradually, educational pursuits became his priority and today he is bilingual, working in international relations in South America. He enjoys recreational activities but respectfully tries to avoid injury.

Participation in organized youth sports has become increasingly popular and widespread over the past several decades. In the United States, 30 to 45 million children and adolescents participate in organized sports each year [1]. Although sport participation promotes an active lifestyle and decreases the risk of childhood obesity, a concern among medical professionals has been the increased pressure for youth to specialize in sports at an early age. Today, it is not uncommon to find young gymnasts and figure skaters training 20-plus hours per week, year round. Similarly, hockey and soccer players as young as 6 years old travel hundreds of miles for competitions. Connected to excessive playing time and overtraining is the increased likelihood of injury.

Injury rates among youth sport participants are high. Sport and exercise related injuries accounted for 65% of emergency department visits surveyed over 1 year for youth under 19 years of age [2]. Although injuries are often minor with respect to time loss [3], stresses associated with injury may be significant, especially for youth experiencing injury for the first time. While the physical components of injury are usually the focus of treatment, the stress associated with injury and recovery may be minimized and escape detection. Without recognition and, on occasion, intervention, psychosocial stressors may precipitate injury and negatively impact rehabilitation and sport performance upon return to the sport.

For the sake of brevity, this article does not focus on physical factors, such as excessive playing time, overtraining, and burnout that influence injury and rehabilitation. Instead the discussion in this article is on psychosocial factors (eg, athletic identity, body image, sport environment, and other social influences, such as life stress) that may impact children and adolescent athletes before and following injury. The article concludes by discussing psychologic interventions that help alleviate stress and total mood disturbance (TMD) resulting from injury.

Athletic injury prediction models

Over the last two decades, two pivotal, empiric sport injury models (Fig. 1) have evolved to investigate psychosocial factors that may influence the risk of obtaining a sport injury and recovery following injury. The Andersen and Williams model (see top portion of Fig. 1) provided a framework to examine psychologic precursors, such as personality, history of stressors, and coping resources in relation to sport injury [4]. The main premise of this model is that a psychophysiologic response is elicited if an athlete cognitively appraises a situation (rational or irrational) as stressful, has a history of stressors, has a personality likely to intensify the stress

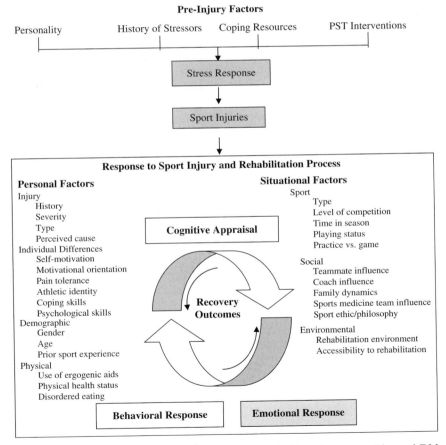

Fig. 1. An integrated model of response to sport injury. (*Adapted from* Wiese-Bjornstal DM, Smith AM, Shaffer SM, et al. An integrated model of response to sport injury: psychologic and sociologic dynamics. J Appl Sport Psychol 1998;10:46–69; with permission from Taylor and Francis Ltd, http://tandf.co.uk/journals.)

response, and has few coping resources. These variables, alone or in combination, precipitate a stress response [4]. Once a stress response is elicited, physiologic and attentional changes occur (ie, increased muscle tension, narrowing of the visual field, and distractibility), thereby increasing likelihood of injury [5].

Wiese-Bjornstal and colleagues (see bottom half of Fig. 1) [6–8] expanded the Andersen and Williams [4] stress injury model by examining emotional response and psychologic recovery following injury. In accordance with the Andersen and Williams model, the stress response associated with personality, history of stressors, and coping, which influence athletes before injury, continues to influence athletes after injury. These same factors, along with the stress of being injured, influence the athlete's ability to cognitively appraise the injury situation. Cognitive appraisal dictates an athlete's emotional reaction to injury that ultimately determines behavioral responses to injury and rehabilitation [6–8]. Furthermore, it is hypothesized that an athlete's cognitive, emotional, and behavioral response to injury is influenced by personal and situational factors. Personal factors that may affect recovery from injury include injury history and severity, motivation to recover from injury, mood state, and coping abilities. Gender, prior sport experience, and use of ergogenic aids are additional personal factors that may influence injury recovery. Situational factors that may potentially affect injury recovery include level of competition, time in season, playing status, and influences from teammates, coaches, and sports medicine professionals. While these factors directly affect the cognitive, emotional, and behavioral response, they indirectly affect physical and psychologic recovery from injury.

Although a complete review of the literature is not warranted for this article, these two injury models highlight physical and psychosocial stressors that may affect injury rates, in addition to injury recovery and after-injury sport performance. Only research on psychosocial stressors relevant to the child, adolescent, and young adulthood populations are thoroughly reviewed in this article.

Psychologic stressors before injury

As postulated by Andersen and Williams (see top portion of Fig. 1) [4], history of stressors (ie, life event stress, daily hassles, and previous injury history), personality characteristics (ie, hardiness, locus of control, and competitive trait anxiety), and coping resources (ie, general coping behaviors, social support, stress management, and psychologic skills training) directly elicit a stress response, while indirectly influencing injury occurrence. Early research in this domain focused on the unidimensional relationships of life event stress, competitive trait anxiety, and social support to injury occurrence. Although all these psychologic variables positively relate to injury occurrence [9–14], life event stress has been the most compelling. Of 35 studies reviewed, 30 related life event stress to sport injury [15]. Furthermore, athletes with high life stress were two to five times more likely to sustain athletic injury [16]. When analyzed by negative and positive life stress, negatively appraised life events were significantly more likely to predict sport injury occurrence [15]. Despite empiric evidence that unidimensional relationships exist between personality, coping resources, and history of stressors to injury, little was known about the moderating effects these variables would have on the life event stress-injury relationship [17].

Petrie [10] examined collegiate female gymnasts and reported that high negative life event stress accounted for 14% to 24% of the injury variance for gymnasts with low levels of social support. No significant life event stress-injury relationship was found among gymnasts with high social support. Smith and colleagues [12] found negative life event stress accounted for 22% to 30% of the injury variance when athletes reported a combination of high stress and low social support and coping ability. Athletes with high social support or high coping resources did not elicit a negative life event-stress injury relationship.

Maddison and Prapavessis [18] studied rugby players (16–34 years of age). Social support, coping resources, competitive trait anxiety, and history of stressors to injury occurrence were examined. Negative life event stress accounted for 31% of the injury variance for rugby players who used avoidance-focused coping behaviors (eg, denial and wishful thinking), who reported having inadequate social support, and had a history of previous injuries. Competitive trait anxiety was not significant. Finally, Rogers and Landers [17] examined the influence of negative life event stress, social support, and coping on sport injury occurrence. A secondary purpose was to examine the role of peripheral narrowing on the life event stress-injury relationship for adolescent soccer players. Negative life event stress and poor coping skills significantly contributed to injury occurrence. Simultaneously, high coping skills buffered the negative life event stress-injury relationship. Peripheral narrowing, influenced by life event stress, increased the likelihood of injury occurrence.

These results support the Anderson and Williams [4] empiric model, indicating that psychologic factors may directly elicit a stress response and indirectly increase the risk of injury for young athletes. Medical professionals should be aware of the influence negative life events have on injury occurrence and be able to help young athletes cope with these events. Given the empiric support for psychologic skill training intervention effect on reducing injury vulnerability [17,18], medical professionals should provide social support, if need be, and teach young athletes skills that will equip them to cope with life event stress. The psychologic interventions section at the end of this article provides specific information on helping athletes cope with psychosocial stressors.

Psychologic stressors following injury

Athletic identity, self-esteem, total mood disturbance

Athletic identity refers to "the degree to which an individual identifies with their athletic role" [19]. Athletes with high athletic identity identify primarily with sport, whereas athletes with a low athletic identity tend to participate in multiple activities, with sport being one of many activities. One benefit of strongly identifying with the athletic role is an increase in self-esteem. For older children and adolescents, high self-esteem helps mediate the continuous physical, psychologic, and social changes that occur during this developmental period [20]. Participation in sport correlates positively with high self-esteem scores [20–22], particularly in the esteem domains of physical appearance and physical competency [20]. Ironically, this same athletic identification that serves to protect self-esteem before injury is a risk factor for diminished feelings of self worth and increased mood disturbance after injury.

Sonestrom and Morgan [23] were the first to examine the impact of injury on a multidimensional measure of self-esteem. Results revealed a post-injury decrease in the physical self-efficacy and perceived physical competency dimensions of self-esteem. These results support the notion that components of self-esteem that protect self-worth before injury also serve to decrease it following an injury. Furthermore, the majority of studies that examined before- and after-injury changes, using a unidimensional measure of self-esteem, found diminished self-esteem after injury [24–28]. McGowan and colleagues [28] conducted in-depth qualitative interviews with injured collegiate football players to examine the reasoning for decreased self-worth after injury. Themes that emerged related to the isolation players felt from their team and the fact that the team was continuing to win without them. These results reveal athletes who sustain an injury also show significant changes to self-esteem after injury. Coupled with diminished self-esteem is an increased risk for total mood disturbance.

Brewer [29] conducted a series of four studies examining the relationship between an athlete's identification with the athlete role to after-injury depression for real and imagined injuries. Results supported his hypothesis that collegiate athletes who identified highly with the athletic role were more likely to respond to an injury with depression. Similarly, adolescent athletes who had a high athletic identity also responded with high depressive symptoms [30]. Moreover, Smith and colleagues [31] studied before- and after-injury mood state and self-esteem changes among competitive high school and collegiate athletes. Results indicated a statistically significant change in total mood disturbance before and after injury. Specifically, before injury the athletes exhibited a positive mental health profile: low levels of depression, anger, confusion, and fatigue, and high levels of vigor. Following injury, the mental health profile reversed, showing high levels of depression and anger, and low levels of vigor. When examined further, the increase in depression was significantly related to the severity of the injury. This finding supported an earlier study conducted by Smith and colleagues [32], in which severity of injury was a significant predictor of depression in injured, recreational athletes.

For most athletes, the increased TMD lasts approximately 1 month [33], with negative mood disturbance occurring immediately following injury and subsiding as the athlete perceives recovery to be occurring [32]. However, for some athletes TMD may not return to before-injury states. Mood disturbance is a concern for adolescent and young adults who are already at approximately three times greater risk for suicide than the general population [34].

Smith and Milliner [33] reported on five case studies in which injured athletes attempted suicide. Common risk factors associated with the attempted suicides included: (1) an injury that required surgery; (2) a long, demanding rehabilitation that prevented athletes from participating in their sport for at least 6 months; (3) a decrease in athletic skills as a result of the injury; (4) little confidence in their ability to perform at before-injury levels following rehabilitation; (5) replacement by a teammate; and (6) experience of substantial success in their sport before the injury.

These case studies highlight the relevancy of research that suggests young athletes who identify highly with a sport and who sustain an injury have an increased risk for diminished self-worth and increased mood disturbance after injury. Most athletes take injury "in stride" [33]. However, some feel so devalued after an injury that depression may reach clinical levels and thoughts of and attempts at taking one's life may occur. During patient assessment, medical professionals should be aware of young athletes' psychologic responses after injury and during the rehabilitation process. Changes in affect, energy, sleep patterns, eye contact, commitment to rehabilitation, and hygiene may be flags for concern. Refer injured athletes to a sport psychologist for counseling for mild to moderate depression and to a sport psychiatrist if depression seems profound (eg, thoughts of suicide, identification of a plan, and acknowledgment of having obtained the means to carry out the plan). Admission for observation and treatment may be indicated.

Body image and eating disorders

Although a review of disordered eating patterns among children and adolescents can be found elsewhere in this issue, this article discusses the impact athletic injury has on the development of eating disorders which can occur in both genders. Young female athletes often have dual, contradicting pressures from society and their athletic participation to satisfy the status quo of an ideal body physique. In Western society, adolescents experience pressure to be thin and have a low body weight. In athletics, female athletes must be strong and muscular, a perception by many that sport is generally associated with masculinity [35]. To offset this perception of masculinity and to conform to the perception of having an ideal body physique, female athletes may resort to unhealthy eating behaviors, such as binging, purging, prolonged fasting, and the use of diuretics, laxatives, and diet pills. Disordered eating and intensive training often leads to the development of the female athlete triad: eating disorder, amenorrhea, and osteoporosis [36–38].

Each of the three disorders can alone or in combination have short and long-term health consequences. Risk increases for musculosketal injuries, such as stress fractures and premature osteoporosis because of a loss in bone mineral density [39]. Athletic injury is one possible explanation for the development of one or a combination of all three triad disorders. Sundgot-Borgen [40] studied trigger factors for the development of anorexia nervosa, bulimia nervosa, and anorexia athletica among elite female Norwegian athletes between the ages of 12 and 35 years. Injury was one of several factors that triggered an eating disorder. The anxiety associated with restriction of physical activity, in combination with the contradictory standards about the ideal body physique [35], performing in aesthetic sports where leanness is a priority, and the pressure placed on athletes by coaches to conform to strict diet plans may place injured athletes at increased risk for an eating disorder. Although more research is needed to verify the role athletic injuries have on the development of one or more of the female athlete triad disorders, medical professionals should watch for signs that the athletic injury may be precipitating an eating disorder. If warranted, the injured athlete should be promptly referred to a comprehensive eating disorder team [41].

Use of ergogenic aids

A serious injury may result in the need for surgery, time away from sports and the team, rehabilitation, an actual or perceived loss of fitness and athletic skill, and a loss in confidence, as well as the possibility of being replaced on the team [33]. Consequently, injured athletes may be tempted to hurry the healing process by using performance enhancing substances, such as steroids, supplements, prescription drugs, or other substances such as stimulants. Initiating a medical program (even though it is a form of drug abuse) may either actually or be perceived to boost performance.

At present, determining the prevalence of drug use in sport and exercise by adolescents is difficult to accurately assess. Detection requires self-reporting or drug testing. Self-reporting is confounded by validity issues. Validity depends on the honesty of a young athlete who would prefer his or her use not be known. Drug testing is expensive and limited by the sophistication of designer steroids, human growth hormones, and masking agents to help athletes escape detection.

To provide a framework to understand drug abuse, Strelan and Boeckmann [42] adapted a deterrence theory, used to assess the likelihood of compliance with the law, to a model for understanding performance-enhancing drug use in elite athletes. This theory is based on the relationship between deterrents or costs versus benefits. For example, deterrents (costs), such as suspensions, disapproval, guilt, reduced self-esteem and health concerns are weighed against benefits, such as prize money, scholarships, acknowledgment, and achievements. Both deterrents and benefits are moderated by sport related situational factors (eg, level of the athlete's participation, type and reputation of the drug, and perceived competitiveness). Because elite athletes serve as powerful role models for younger athletes, it is likely that similar processes occur in aspiring adolescents. Adolescent injured athletes are often vulnerable, depressed, deconditioned, and unable to participate in sports, as discussed earlier. The signed preseason contract stating that the young athlete would not use alcohol or drugs during the athletic season has become a moot point and substance abuse may seem like the only way back [43]. Physicians and other health care professionals, in prescribing responsibly, may help prevent substance abuse in injured athletes.

According to the Office of National Drug Control Policy, physicians were the source for 18.3% of narcotics being used by teenagers. The remaining adolescents obtained prescription pain medications from parents, peers, or relatives, perhaps by stealing them from medicine cabinets (10.2%) [44]. Because surgical procedures in adolescents may occur more often for sport-related injuries than for other medical problems, becoming a major source of prescription drugs is a concern for sports medicine practitioners. In addition to health care professionals, other sources include the Internet and workout gyms.

The use of performance enhancing drugs or the abuse of prescription drugs is illegal, immoral, and dangerous. Furthermore, it usually escalates, is expensive, and most often has a negative effect on the athlete's health [45]. Unfortunately, the solution to the problem is as difficult and multifaceted as the problem itself.

Concluding comments

As postulated by Wiese-Bjornstal and colleagues [6], when young athletes become injured, personal stressors can affect how they respond and how quickly they recover following an injury. For example, when identity and self-worth is completely accounted for by sport, injury may result in athletes asking: "If I'm not an athlete, then who am I?" This identity crisis [46] negatively affects feelings of self-worth and contributes to TMD. For some athletes, the feelings associated with not being able to participate in sport and exercise may result in risk taking behaviors, including unhealthy eating patterns, suicidal ideations, and drug use to substitute for the athletic "high." For other athletes, dealing with the physical pain of injury is easier to cope with than dealing with the emotional pain of isolation and depression. For some of these athletes, continuing to train and compete through injury may be perceived as their only viable option; thus, they may return to sport prematurely.

Sociologic stressors following injury

Along with personal factors, situational factors such as level of competition (eg, varsity versus junior varsity), time in season (eg, beginning versus end of season), playing status (eg, starter versus nonstarter), and perceived role on the team may also affect injured athletes' cognitive appraisal and emotional response to injury. If athletes perceive the injury to be a threat to their position and status on the team or to their ability to compete in upcoming competitions, they may ignore medical advice and the physical pain of injury and accept the "culture of risk" [47]. In the culture of risk, training and competing through injury is acceptable and encouraged.

Sport environmental factors

In a study examining the reasoning for why high school gymnasts continue to train and compete despite injury, gymnasts reported that older, varsity level gymnasts were more likely to train through injury to ensure their position on the team was maintained and to retain current skill levels. The ultimate goal was to be able to compete at the state competition at the end of the season. For these gymnasts, timing of the injury reflected their likelihood of seeking medical advice. Of these gymnasts, 76% indicated they would avoid telling a medical professional of their injury because of fear of the medical "restrictions" ordered as a component of their treatment (Nippert, unpublished doctoral dissertation, 2005).

Podlog and Eklund [48] reported similar results with respect to time in the season and desire to maintain a position on the team. They examined competitive athletes and their return to sports following a serious injury. One injured athlete interviewed commented: "At the end of the year with finals coming up, you're going to sacrifice more than what you would at the start of the season and 99% of people would say the same thing." An injured athlete in a different study validated this finding; "...I think for a lot of players, if it's the last straw, the last chance, it's a whole new motivation. There's a whole new reason to suck it up...." [49].

Perceived role on the team and risk of losing collegiate scholarship opportunities are additional sociologic stressors that may affect how an injured athlete responds to an injury. Fischer, in an unpublished component of a larger published study [50], examined predictors of college scholarship awards for Junior A ice hockey players. Perceived role on the team affected athletes and their prevalence of injury. One 19-year-old defenseman sustained 15 injuries over the season. He perceived that his coaches and teammates expected him to be "a bit mean." He justified his injuries as "it's just my role," although unfortunately several of the injuries were concussions. This case illustrates the significance of cognitive appraisal on injury. Sustaining an injury showed his aggressiveness and, by not taking time off to heal, he was reinforcing that he was playing his role on the team well. To reinforce this perceived role, he was offered a collegiate scholarship to play hockey. One can only speculate whether he would have received a collegiate scholarship if he had stopped playing when injured.

Sportnet influences

Nixon [51] hypothesized that members of an athlete's social support system or "sportnet" contributes to a young athlete's interpretation, support, and coping with pain and injury. Although these individuals usually provide positive support for young athletes when faced with an injury, alternatively they may also negatively encourage athletes to continue training through an injury based upon their own predefined pain and injury beliefs. For children and adolescents, the individuals most likely to be involved in the sportnet include parents, coaches, teammates, and sports medicine professionals.

Parents and coaches

Parents and coaches are the individuals that young athletes turn to first for support and encouragement following an injury. Usually, these significant others provide positive support and encouragement as they contemplate what to do after an injury. Occasionally, however, parents and coaches allow their own pre-existing beliefs about pain and injury to influence a young athlete's response to injury and behavior.

Shaffer (Shaffer, unpublished doctoral dissertation, 1996) interviewed 19 adolescent wrestlers to examine their motivation to wrestle with pain. Results indicated parents and coaches showed both positive and negative reactions to injury. Quotes, such as "my parents just told me that now I have to work harder to get what I want" (p. 72) and "coach pressured me to sit out and rest ... he cared about me and not the points" (p. 70) were expressed by some of the wrestlers. Predominantly, however, the wrestlers felt coaches and parents expressed negative reactions to their injury, pressuring them to return to the sport despite injury. Comments, such as "I didn't have a very good coach. He told me to 'suck up the pain'" (p. 71) and "my dad didn't feel [the injury] was that bad. He's had five knee surgeries and I think he really wanted me back wrestling..." (p. 74) speak volumes to young athletes about what is acceptable behavior when injured. Curry [52] reported that an amateur wrestler's "motivation to achieve excellence" was related to his earliest memories of getting injured when his father "showed no emotional reaction and claimed [injuries were] not significant."

Unique to parents of elite adolescent athletes is the financial and family strain associated with training opportunities. Many training facilities for elite level athletes are located in only a few locations across the country.

For parents, this often requires splitting up the family and working multiple jobs to pay for training costs. This high price for allowing a child to train away from home may contribute to feelings a parent has of being highly invested in their child's training and future success. When an injury occurs, the elite level athlete may feel compelled to continue training despite the injury because of the investment and sacrifice the parents have made. Likewise, because parents have invested so much in the child's future sport success, they may expect their child to train through injury.

Based on societal pressure to win, coaches may prioritize winning as most important and consider the athlete's health as a secondary concern [53]. Veerger and Hogg [54] reported that coaches were significantly more likely to allow a gymnast to compete if she was the best on the team, was older, if the injury was of moderate severity, and if it was a qualifying meet. Many coaches of young athletes have a dual role of coach and medical advisor. This dual role may result in added pressure to young athletes to return to the sport earlier than necessary.

Teammates

For many athletes, teammates are their best friends and serve as a source of social support in and out of sports. When injured, athletes have reported feeling guilty, frustrated, alienated, lonely, and sad over letting their team down and not having daily social contact with their teammates [48,55,56]. Coupled with these feelings is the expectation teammates may have for injured athletes to continue training and competing.

> "...we made a commitment to be on the team and to compete and that as a member of the team you don't back off. I mean it's like you made the commitment, and if you're on varsity, by not giving everything that you have in practice and in meets you're letting the entire team down, you're letting the team score down, and if you don't give everything that you have and the team loses, who's going to feel responsible? I mean the girls who gave it everything or the one who slacked off and just sat there?" (Nippert, unpublished doctoral dissertation, 2005).

This quote highlights an unconditional embracing of the culture of risk for a group of high school gymnasts. According to this teammate, being a member of a team requires a full commitment and sacrifice. By stopping sport participation, injured athletes face resentment from teammates, as they are viewed as not being fully committed to the team. To counteract the feelings of isolation and guilt associated with letting their teammates down, some young athletes may choose health-compromising behaviors.

Medical professionals

Medical professionals generally promote a full recovery from injury before allowing injured athletes to return to full sport participation. Theoretically, diagnosing and providing advice to injured athletes is conducted in an objective setting with no outside influences. Flint and Weiss [53] found that, unlike coaches, athletic trainers were not influenced by game or player status and, thus, were less likely to return a player to a game when injured. Conversely, Safai [49] reported that sports medicine clinicians are influenced by, and influence, a culture where playing through injury and pain is acceptable.

For many clinicians interviewed, time in season, important competitions, and status on the team (ie, starter versus benchwarmer) were factors that contributed to a decision to return an injured athlete. For other clinicians, personal experiences of training and competing with their own injuries influenced them in their negotiations with injured athletes. Thus, although theoretically medical professionals are the least likely members of the sportnet to pressure injured athletes back to sport participation, their decisions and negotiations with the injured athlete also often encompasses a culture of risk. Strauss and Lanese [57] reported that sports medicine staff, working a wrestling camp, indicated 9 to 14 year olds "over-reported" muscle strains and contusions, injuries that older wrestlers worked through. This finding suggests that again a culture of risk permeates societal thinking and medical professionals are not immune to this influence. To ensure objectivity in decision making, medical professionals should be aware of the influence "culture of risk" may have on their decisions with injured athletes.

Concluding comments

Situational factors, such as time in season, playing status, and influences from sportnet individuals affect how athletes respond to an injury. If athletes believe the injury is threatening their position on the team, or if significant others perceive they are faking the injury or are feeling pressured to return to sport earlier, they are not likely to adhere to the complete rehabilitation program and will return to sport early.

Psychosocial stressors affecting sport performance

When injured, athletes have two viable options: stop sport participation and complete procedures, treatment, and rehabilitation in entirety, or return to sport prematurely. Research has demonstrated the role of psychosocial stressors on young athletes as they contemplate injury response. Risk factors for early return to sport include long-term physical pain, which consequently may affect performance, and long-term exercise participation following retirement from sports.

Wadley and Albright [58] examined residual effects of overuse injuries on intercollegiate female gymnasts following retirement from gymnastics. Forty five percent of gymnasts reported injuries sustained during their competitive gymnastics years still bothered them 3 years later. Furthermore, 29% of gymnasts reported limited physical activity because of the reoccurrence of prior injury symptoms aggravated by physical activity. A secondary risk of early return to sports relates to early termination or retirement from sport because of a secondary injury, fear of reinjury, or an incomplete rehabilitation. As a result of these risk factors and psychosocial stress on some injured athletes, ideally medical professionals consider both the physical and psychologic aspects of injury. Psychologic interventions, such as goal setting, relaxation and mental imagery, positive self-talk, and application of attribution theory theoretically and clinically help injured athletes cope.

Psychologic interventions

Abraham Maslow theorized that individuals seek to satisfy fundamental basic human needs. Needs are based on a hierarchal pyramid, with physiologic needs having the highest priority, followed by safety, love and belonging, self-esteem, and self-actualization. When injury occurs, the basic needs of safety, love and belonging, and self-esteem are threatened. Psychologic interventions can help injured athletes reclaim their basic needs, while simultaneously increasing self-esteem and dealing with TMD after injury.

Johnson [59] studied injured competitive athletes with long-term injuries to examine the effect stress management, cognitive control, goal setting, and relaxation or guided imagery had on mood levels. Results revealed that a combination of these psychologic interventions elevated mood states during and at the end of rehabilitation for injured athletes. Similarly, Ievleva and Orlick [60] retrospectively examined slow and fast healing athletes and found the faster healing athletes used psychologic strategies, such as goal setting, positive self-talk, and healing imagery more often during rehabilitation.

From a theoretic standpoint, these results suggest psychologic interventions can elevate mood and improve recovery time following injury. From a clinical perspective, these interventions have been used extensively with injured athletes in a sports medicine facility where the first author worked as a Johannson-Gund Scholar and where the second author counsels. Because the clinical outcomes support the theoretical outcomes, the emphasis on these interventions pertains to the clinical relevancy of actually using the interventions, rather than providing theoretic support for the interventions.

Goal setting

When injury occurs, setting short- and long-term goals is a positive first step toward healing. Medical professionals should work with injured athletes to redirect their sport goals to rehabilitation goals. This is important for children and adolescent athletes who may be experiencing injury for the first time and who may not be aware of goals that must be accomplished during rehabilitation [61]. To set rehabilitation goals, medical professionals can use the target model (Fig. 2), which represents short, intermediate, and

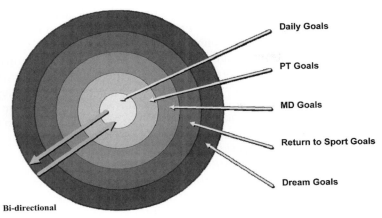

Daily Goals

PT Goals

MD Goals

Return to Sport Goals

Dream Goals

Bi-directional

Fig. 2. Goal setting target model. (*Adapted from* Smith AM. Power play: mental toughness for hockey and beyond. Flagler Beach, FL: Athletic Guide Publishing, 1999; with permission.)

long-term rehabilitation and sport goals. The outer ring of the target reflects the injured athlete's long-term dream sport goal, whereas the inner ring or bull's eye reflects daily rehabilitation goals. This visual target reminds injured athletes that to be successful and meet the long-term dream sport goal, daily rehabilitation goals must be accomplished first. By focusing on daily rehabilitation goals (eg, icing, elevation, flexion, extension, and pain management), and then meeting specified goals of the physical therapist and physician, return to sport goals will be realized.

When setting goals, medical professionals should use the standard of "who will do what by when" [8] to ensure goals are specific and measurable. When a goal is achieved, medical professionals should acknowledge success to enhance motivation and adherence to rehabilitation. Because goals are dynamic, medical professionals should explain that physical and psychologic set-backs will occur during rehabilitation [61]. Consequently, athletes need to re-evaluate goals periodically.

Relaxation and mental imagery

Research has positively supported the use of relaxation and mental imagery for athletes rehabilitating from injury [60,62,63]. Benefits include controlling anxiety and arousal, enhancing pain management, decreasing muscle tension, increasing self-confidence, and enhancing sport performance following recovery [64,65]. Despite the benefits, some injured athletes fail to make the connection that the psychologic strategies used to enhance sport performance will also enhance injury recovery [64]. Ideally, medical professionals should make injured athletes aware of the benefits and purposes of using mental imagery and relaxation for injury rehabilitation [63].

Driediger and colleagues [62] conducted a qualitative analysis on mental imagery use by injured athletes and reported imagery was used for injury recovery and sport performance enhancement. During recovery, imagery is used before executing rehabilitation exercises, for sustaining motivation and focus during a long and often painful rehabilitation, in helping to control stress associated with injury, and increasing feelings of self-efficacy and mental toughness. Finally, injured athletes reported using healing imagery (ie, imagining physiologic tissue repair) to aid in recovery. Specific to sport training, mental imagery is used to execute sport skills and to visualize being fully healed and back competing.

Preoperatively, patients in the sports medicine clinic referred to earlier are guided through a short relaxation script to reduce muscle tension before procedures, such as anterior cruciate ligament reconstruction. Through deep, focused breathing, injured athletes are asked to clear their minds of negative thinking and distractions before moving on to progressively tensing and relaxing major muscle groups in their body [32]. Following the relaxation exercise, injured athletes are instructed in how to use the relaxation technique preoperatively, to enhance the effectiveness of pain medication and before rehabilitation flexion and extension exercises. Finally, athletes practice pairing the expiration phase of deep breathing with the flexion phase of range of motion. Given the breadth of situations in which injured athletes have reported using mental imagery, medical professionals may wish to discuss other scenarios in which imagery can help facilitate injury recovery and sport performance following return to sport. Desensitization to fear of reinjury is an example.

Cognitive restructuring and positive self-talk

Cognitive restructuring and positive self-talk are two psychologic interventions injured athletes can use to get rid of negative, irrational thoughts often associated with injury. Channel clicking [66] is a cognitive restructuring technique that encourages injured athletes to "switch off" their negative, irrational thoughts. When switching the negative thinking channel, injured athletes have two channel options: the positive channel or the imagery channel. If injured athletes are able to successfully restructure their negative "stinkin thinkin" to a positive statement, the switch is made to the positive channel. If a positive switch is not possible, injured athletes are instructed to switch to the imagery channel where positive images (eg, heroes, themselves succeeding, and so forth) can be visualized.

Causal attributions

Attribution theory focuses on explanations for events and behaviors. Possible explanations can be categorized into one or more of the following categories: stability (stable or unstable), locus of causality (internal or

Internal	External	
ABILITY	TASK	Stable
EFFORT	LUCK	Unstable

Fig. 3. Attributions. (*Adapted from* Smith AM. Power play: mental toughness for hockey and beyond. Flagler Beach, FL: Athletic Guide Publishing, 1999; with permission.)

external), and locus of control (in one's control or out of one's control) (Fig. 3) [67]. Each dimension has implications toward behavior. For example, injured athletes who make stable attributes expect the same outcome to occur again, whereas unstable attributions lead to expectations of different outcomes in the future. Moreover, internal attributes (ie, talent or ability) increases pride and shame, while external attributes (ie, luck, weather) decreases these feelings. Finally, controllability factors increase or decrease motivation depending upon whether the injured athlete perceives injury to be within or outside of their control.

When injury occurs, what athletes attribute their injury to may affect rehabilitation and injury recovery. Injured athletes who perceive rehabilitation and recovery to be internal, stable, and within their control are more likely to comply with rehabilitation. In contrast, injured athletes who attribute recovery to factors that are unstable and not within their control are less likely to adhere to rehabilitation [68,69]. This denial will affect injury recovery.

These results draw attention to the importance of monitoring and correcting inappropriate attributes that injured athletes may make about their injury. When making corrections, Weinberg and Gould [70] suggest linking attributes to individual goals and capabilities as well as to one's ability and effort.

Summary

This article addressed the impact psychosocial stressors have on injury recovery and the sport performance of young injured athletes. Medical professionals aware of psychosocial stressors unique to young athletes that may contribute to injury occurrence and influence rehabilitation, may help counter the negative effects and unhealthy behavioral responses that sometimes occur post-injury. Through awareness and appropriate interventions, medical professionals can help facilitate an optimal physical and psychologic recovery.

Acknowledgment

The authors thank Dr. Eric Milliner, an adolescent sport psychiatrist from the Mayo Clinic, for his years of experience working with adolescent athletes. Dr. Milliner uses medication only when needed. Thankfully, most patients leave his office feeling better about themselves and their sports.

References

[1] Brenner JS. Overuse injuries, overtraining, and burnout in child and adolescent athletes. Pediatrics 2007;119(6):1242–5.

[2] Centers for Disease Control and Prevention. Morbidity and mortality weekly report: non-fatal sports-and recreation-related injuries treated in emergency departments, United States, July 2000–June 2001. Morbidity and Mortality Weekly Report 2002;51(33):736–9. Available at: http://www.cdc.gov/mmwr/preview/mmwrhtml/mm5133a2.htm. Accessed July 2, 2007.

[3] Caine D, Caine C, Maffulli N. Incidence and distribution of pediatric sport-related injuries. Clin J Sport Med 2006;16:500–13.

[4] Andersen MB, Williams JM. A model of stress and athletic injury: prediction and prevention. J Sport Exerc Psychol 1988;10:294–306.

[5] Williams JM, Andersen MB. Psychosocial antecedents of sport injury: review and critique of the stress and injury model. Journal of Applied Sport Psychology 1998;10:5–25.

[6] Wiese-Bjornstal DM, Smith AM, Shaffer SM, et al. An integrated model of response to sport injury: psychological and sociological dynamics. Journal of Applied Sport Psychology 1998; 10:46–69.

[7] Wiese-Bjornstal DM, Smith AM, LaMott EE. A model of psychologic response to athletic injury and rehabilitation. Athletic training: Sports Health Care Perspectives 1995;1(1): 17–30.

[8] Wiese DM, Weiss MS. Psychological rehabilitation and physical injury: implications for the sportsmedicine team. The Sport Psychologist 1987;1:318–30.

[9] Patterson EL, Smith RE, Everett JJ, et al. Interactive effects of life stress as predictors of ballet injuries. Journal of Sport Behavior 1998;21:101–12.

[10] Petrie TA. Psychosocial antecedents of athletic injury: the effects of life stress and social support on female collegiate gymnasts. Behav Med 1992;18:127–38.

[11] Petrie TA. Coping skills, competitive trait anxiety, and playing status: moderating effects of the life stress-injury relationship. J Sport Exerc Psychol 1993;15:261–74.

[12] Smith RE, Smoll FL, Ptacek JT. Conjunctive moderator variables in vulnerability and resiliency research: life stress, social support, and coping skills, and adolescent sport injuries. J Pers Soc Psychol 1990;58:360–9.

[13] Hanson SJ, McCullagh P, Tonymon P. The relationship of personality characteristics, life stress, and coping resources to athletic injury. J Sport Exerc Psychol 1992;14:262–72.

[14] Williams JM, Tonymon P, Wadsworth WA. Relationship of stress to injury in intercollegiate volleyball. J Human Stress 1986;12:38–43.

[15] Williams JM. Psychology of injury risk and prevention. In: Singer RN, Hausenblas HA, Janelle CM, editors. Handbook of sport psychology. 2nd edition. New York: J Wiley; 2001. p. 766–86.

[16] Williams JM, Roepke N. Psychology of injury and injury rehabilitation. In: Singer RN, Tennant LK, Murphey M, editors. Handbook of research on sport psychology. New York: Macmillan; 1993. p. 815–39.

[17] Rogers TJ, Landers DM. Mediating effects of peripheral vision in the life event stress/athletic injury relationship. J Sport Exerc Psychol 2005;27:271–88.

[18] Maddison R, Prapavessis H. A psychological approach to the prediction and prevention of athletic injury. J Sport Exerc Psychol 2005;27:289–310.

[19] Brewer B, Van Raalte J, Linder D. Athletic identity: Hercules' muscles or Achilles heel? Int J Sport Psychol 1993;24:237–54.

[20] Bowker A. The relationship between sports participation and self-esteem during early adolescence. Can J Behav Sci 2006;38(3):214–29.

[21] Koivula N. Sport participation: differences in motivation and actual participation due to gender typing. Journal of Sport Behavior 1999;22:360–81.

[22] Taylor D. A comparison of college athletic participants and nonparticipants on self-esteem. Journal of College Student Development 1995;36:444–51.

[23] Sonestrom RJ, Morgan WP. Exercise and self-esteem: rationale and model. Med Sci Sports Exerc 1989;21:329–37.

[24] Chan CS, Grossman HY. Psychological effects of running loss on consistent runners. Percept Mot Skills 1988;66:875–83.

[25] Kolt GS, Roberts PDT. Self-esteem and injury in competitive field hockey players. Percept Mot Skills 1998;87:353–4.

[26] Tracey J. The emotional response to the injury and rehabilitation process. Journal of Applied Sport Psychology 2003;15:279–93.

[27] Leddy MH, Lambert MJ, Ogles BM. Psychological consequences of athletic injury among high-level competitors. Res Q Exerc Sport 1994;65(4):347–54.

[28] McGowan RW, Pierce EF, Williams M, et al. Athletic injury and self-diminution. J Sports Med Phys Fitness 1994;34:299–304.

[29] Brewer BW. Self-identity and specific vulnerability to depressed mood. J Pers 1993;61(3): 343–64.

[30] Manuel JC, Shilt JS, Curl WW, et al. Coping with sports injuries: an examination of the adolescent athlete. J Adolesc Health 2002;31:391–3.

[31] Smith AM, Stuart MJ, Wiese-Bjornstal DM, et al. Competitive athletes: preinjury and post-injury mood state and self-esteem. Mayo Clin Proc 1993;68:939–47.

[32] Smith AM, Scott SG, O'Fallon WM, et al. Emotional responses of athletes to injury. Mayo Clin Proc 1990;65:38–50.

[33] Smith AM, Milliner EK. Injured athletes and the risk of suicide. J Athl Train 1994;29(4): 337–41.

[34] Sabo D, Miller KE, Melnick MJ, et al. High school athletic participation and adolescent suicide: a nationwide US study. International Review for the Sociology of Sport 2005; 40(1):5–23.

[35] Crissey SR, Honea JC. The relationship between athletic participation and perceptions of body size and weight control in adolescent girls: the role of sport type. Sociol Sport J 2006;23:248–72.

[36] Torstveit MK, Sundgot-Borgen J. The female athlete triad: are elite athletes at increased risk? Med Sci Sports Exerc 2005;37:184–93.

[37] Otis CL, Drinkwater B, Johnson A, et al. American College of Sports Medicine position stand. The female athlete triad. Med Sci Sports Exerc 1997;29:i–ix.

[38] Yeager KK, Agostini R, Nattiv A, et al. The female athlete triad: disordered eating, amenorrhea, osteoporosis. Med Sci Sports Exerc 1993;25:775–7.

[39] Hobart JA, Smucker DR. The female athlete triad. Am Fam Physician 2000;61(11):3357–70. Available at: http://www.aafp.org/afp/20000601/3357.html. Accessed July 24, 2007.

[40] Sundgot-Borgen J. Risk and trigger factors for the development of eating disorders in female elite athletes. Med Sci Sports Exerc 1994;26:414–9.

[41] Beals K. Disordered eating among athletes: a comprehensive guide for health professionals. Illinois (IL): Human Kinetics; 2004.

[42] Strelan P, Boeckmann RJ. A new model for understanding performance-enhancing drug use by elite athletes. Journal of Applied Sport Psychology 2003;15(2):176–83.

[43] Rosengren J. Blades of glory: The true story of a young team bred to win. Naperville, IL: Sourcebooks, Inc.; 2003.

[44] Teens and prescription drugs. An analysis of recent trends on the emerging drug threat. Office of National Drug Control Policy 2007. Available at: http://www.mediacampaign. org/teens/brochure.pdf. Accessed August 21, 2007.

[45] Pipe A, Ayotte C. Nutritional supplements and doping. Clin J Sport Med 2002;12(4): 245–9.

[46] Stephan Y, Brewer BW. Perceived determinants of identification with the athlete role among elite competitors. Journal of Applied Sport Psychology 2007;19:67–79.

[47] Nixon HL. Coaches' views of risk, pain, and injury in sport, with special reference to gender differences. Sociol Sport J 1994;11:79–87.

[48] Podlog L, Eklund RC. A longitudinal investigation of competitive athletes' return to sport following serious injury. Journal of Applied Sport Psychology 2006;18:44–68.

[49] Safai P. Healing the body in the "culture of risk": examining the negotiation of treatment between sport medicine clinicians and injured athletes in Canadian intercollegiate sport. Sociol Sport J 2003;20:127–46.

[50] Stuart MJ, Smith AM, Malo-Ortiguera SA, et al. A comparison of facial protection and the incidence of head, neck, and facial injuries in Junior A hockey players: a function of individual playing time. Am J Sports Med 2002;30(1):39–44.

[51] Nixon HL. A social network analysis of influences on athletes to play with pain and injury. Journal of Sport and Social Issues 1992;16:127–35.

[52] Curry T. A little pain never hurt anyone: athletic career socialization and the normalization of sports injury. Symbolic Interaction 1993;16:273–90.

[53] Flint FA, Weiss MR. Returning injured athletes to competition: a role and ethical dilemma. Can J Sport Sci 1992;17:34–40.

[54] Vergeer I, Hogg JM. Coaches' decision policies about the participation of injured athletes in competition. The Sport Psychologist 1999;13:42–56.

[55] Cassidy CM. Understanding sport-injury anxiety. Athletic Therapy Today 2006;11(4):57–8.

[56] Wrisberg CA, Fisher LA. Staying connected to teammates during rehabilitation. Athletic Therapy Today 2005;10(2):62–3.

[57] Strauss RH, Lanese RR. Injuries among wrestlers in school and college tournaments. JAMA 1982;284:2016–9.

[58] Wadley GH, Albright JP. Women's intercollegiate gymnastics. Injury patterns and "permanent" medical disability. Am J Sports Med 1993;21:314–20.

[59] Johnson U. Short-term psychological intervention: a study of long-term-injured competitive athletes. J Sport Rehabil 2000;9:207–18.

[60] Ievleva L, Orlick T. Mental links to enhanced healing: an exploratory study. The Sport Psychologist 1991;5:25–40.

[61] Wayda VK, Armenth-Brothers F, Boyce AB. Goal setting: a key to injury rehabilitation. Athletic Therapy Today 1998;3(1):21–5.

[62] Driediger M, Hall C, Callow N. Imagery use by injured athletes: a qualitative analysis. J Sports Sci 2006;24(3):261–71.

[63] Green LB. The use of imagery in the rehabilitation of injured athletes. The Sport Psychologist 1992;6:416–28.

[64] Sordoni C, Hall C, Forwell L. The use of imagery by athletes during injury rehabilitation. J Sport Rehabil 2000;9:329–38.

[65] Wiese-Bjornstal DM, Smith AM. Counseling strategies for enhanced recovery of injured athletes within a team approach. In: Pargman D, editor. Psychological bases of sports injuries. Morgantown (WV): Fitness Information Technology; 1993. p. 149–82.

[66] Orlick T. Reflections on sportspych consulting with individual and team sport athletes at Summer and Winter olympic games. Sport Psychologist 1989;3:358–65.

[67] Weiner B. An attribution theory of motivation and emotion. New York: Springer-Verlag; 1986.

[68] Brewer BW, Cornelius AE, Van Raalte JL, et al. Attributions for recovery and adherence to rehabilitation following anterior cruciate ligament reconstruction: a prospective analysis. Psychol Health 2000;15:283–91.

[69] Grove JR, Hanrahan SJ, Stewart RM. Attributions for rapid or slow recovery from sports injuries. Can J Sport Sci 1990;15:107–14.

[70] Weinberg RS, Gould D. Motivation. In: Weinberg RS, Gould D, editors. Foundations of sport and exercise psychology. 4th edition. (IL): Human Kinetics; 2007. p. 51–76.

ELSEVIER
SAUNDERS

Phys Med Rehabil Clin N Am
19 (2008) 419–427

PHYSICAL MEDICINE
AND REHABILITATION
CLINICS OF
NORTH AMERICA

Index

Note: Page numbers of article titles are in **boldface** type.